An Eye Doctor Answers

Explanations To Hundreds Of The Most Common Questions Patients Wish They Had Asked

Richard A. Driscoll, O.D.

Physician's Publishing Group

This book is not intended to substitute for the medical advice of your doctor. The reader should consult with his or her doctor with regard to all matters relating to his or her health.

Copyright © 2012 by Richard A. Driscoll, O.D.

Cover Design by: Radoslaw Krawczyk

ISBN: 0984847200 (Paperback)
ISBN-13: 978-0-9848472-0-4 (Paperback)
ISBN-13: 978-0-9848472-4-2 (Kindle eBook)
ISBN-13: 978-0-9848472-5-9 (EPUB)

v2012.09.261708

DEDICATION

To my family Diana, Taylor, and Jimmie--you mean the world to me. And to my parents, Cloe and Judy Driscoll, I could not have better role models.

TABLE OF CONTENTS

ADDENDUM

ACKNOWLEDGMENT

Writing a book is something I have wanted to do for a long time and I am truly grateful to all of those people who have helped move this project from ideas in my head to something people could finally hold in their hand. I appreciate the help and encouragement I have received from so many people who have made this possible. A few people, however, have been particularly instrumental in seeing this projection to completion.

I'd like to thank my wife, Dr. Diana Driscoll, not only for her encouragement and advice, but also for letting me publish in this book the excellent sections she wrote on the ocular complications of Ehlers-Danlos Syndrome. I'd also like to thank Dr. Alycia Green for her technical editing of the manuscript. This book is filled with hundreds of facts. Your help was invaluable not only in making sure I got the details right, but I appreciated all of your other suggestions as well. Last, I'd like to say thanks to Mr. Dale Schmeltzle, the author of *Highly Visible Marketing: 115 Low-cost Ways to Avoid Market Obscurity,* for encouraging me to stop thinking about writing a book and actually do it. Thank you so much, everyone.

Dr. Richard A Driscoll

FOREWORD

When I first started to write this book, I set out to answer the fifty most common questions asked of eye doctors. It soon became apparent that in the almost 25 years I have been seeing patients, I have answered a lot more questions than I realized. My list began to rapidly grow. In the pages that follow, I answer almost 400 of the most common eye questions and, where relevant, I have also provided the references to my statements.

My intent in writing this book was to answer the most common eye care questions as if you, the reader, were sitting in the exam room with me. Therefore, I have written this book in a conversational style as if we were talking together.

I find that most doctors, myself included of course, like it when patients ask questions. We want our patients to understand what we are talking about and be a partner in our patients medical care. Patients should never be afraid to let their doctor know that they don't understand what the doctor is saying.

At the end of my exam, I'll present to my patient what we have found and how I suggest we treat the condition.

I'll then ask, "Do you have any more questions?"

Frequently, they will say "Yes, but I just can't remember it."

"Okay," I'll tell them "if you think of it later call me or write it down and bring it with you next time."

You can imagine what happens. Rarely does someone call, and even less often does anyone write their question down and bring it with them next time. This was essentially the impetus behind this book; I wanted to find a way for patients to get answers to those questions they forgot to ask.

We all know a picture is worth a thousand words, thus I have included many images and illustrations throughout the book. For those who want to see the color version of these images, there is also a full color electronic version of this book. The eBook, of course, has all of the color images and can be read using a Kindle or iPad. If you don't have an eReader yet Amazon also makes the electronic version available for viewing online via your PC.

The addendum on *The Ocular Complications of Ehlers-Danlos Syndrome* and *What are the Ocular Symptoms of Ehlers-Danlos Syndrome* was written by my wife, Dr. Diana Driscoll, which is an excellent guide for patients and doctors who wish to know more about the ocular complications of Ehlers-Danlos Syndrome. Much more information on not only Ehlers-Danlos, but also conditions such as MS, Chronic Fatigue, Lyme Disease, and Fibromyalgia can be found on her website, www.Prettyill.com.

When referring to doctors, I have interchangeably used he/she or him/her throughout the book. At the back of the book you will find an index to make it easier to quickly find answers to your questions. However, if you don't see the answer to the question you have always wanted to know, feel free to submit your question on The Eye Doc Blog www.TheEyeDocBlog.com and I'll try to answer your question online or in the next edition.

Thanks for reading the book. I hope you will find it helpful in your quest to learn more about your healthcare.

Richard A. Driscoll, O.D.
Dallas/Ft. Worth, Texas
December 2011

An Eye Doctor Answers

*Explanations To Hundreds Of
The Most Common Questions
Patients Wish They Had Asked*

Richard A. Driscoll, O.D.

Physician's Publishing Group

HOW TO GET THE MOST OUT OF THIS BOOK

To answer questions about the eye it is best to lead off with a brief lesson on ocular anatomy, therefore I placed this at the front of the book. Questions are organized based on the eye's anatomy, starting with the eyelids and ending with the optic nerve and retina.

Most questions, but not all, are easy to categorize this way so like almost everything there are a few exceptions. The most common questions asked of eye doctors are always related to the types of refractive errors such as, what is nearsightedness, what is astigmatism, etc., therefore Chapter Two answers questions about refractive errors.

Many questions such as those related to children's vision and vision therapy deserve their own category. And of course, there is a miscellaneous section.

A list of all of the questions in this book can be found on page 225. This book also has an extensive index which begins on page 238. There are numerous black and white photos and diagrams in this book. If you would like to see these photographs in color I invite you to download the eBook version which can also be read on a personal computer.

I've answered the most common questions in *An Eye Doctor Answers*; however, I continue to hear good questions that aren't in the book and would be good additions. If you don't see your question here please visit us on www.TheEyeDocBlog.com and feel free to submit your question on the blog. You may find your answer in a future blog post or an in a new edition.

Thanks for reading and I hope you find what you are looking for.

Dr. Richard A Driscoll

CHAPTER ONE

Ocular Anatomy

Before we start answering any other questions about the eye we should first get an understanding of basic eye anatomy. The eye is connected to the brain via the optic nerve. The optic nerve is not really a true nerve, but an extension of the brain. The optic nerve is the second cranial nerve. The eye is the only place on the body where we can directly see arteries and veins without surgery. Did you know you can actually determine one's pulse while looking into the eye with an ophthalmoscope?

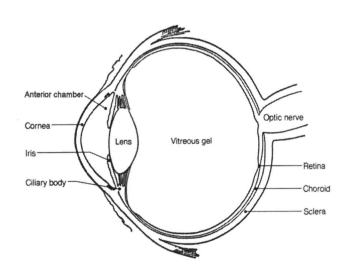

Figure 1   Cross Section of Eye

Many questions fielded by eye doctors naturally revolve around vision correction and the many different ways a patient's vision can be modified, therefore it is important to understand the corneal anatomy.

In the Figure 2, the bottom layer is known as the corneal endothelium. Its purpose is to maintain corneal clarity. The next layer up from the bottom is the corneal stroma. As you can see, the stroma makes up the majority of the corneal thickness and gives the cornea its strength. Bowman's membrane is the next layer, followed by the outermost layer of the cornea, the corneal epithelium.

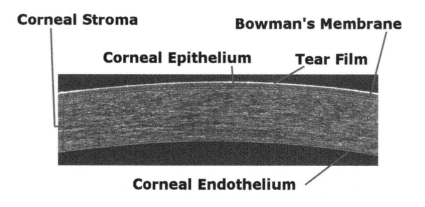

Figure 2   High Resolution Optical Coherence Tomography of the Cornea

CHAPTER TWO

Refractive Conditions

Hands down, the most common questions asked of eye doctors are related to the various refractive conditions; nearsightedness (myopia), farsightedness (hyperopia), astigmatism, and presbyopia.

Nearsightedness

What is Nearsightedness?

Myopia, or nearsightedness, is a condition where a person's uncorrected vision is only clear up close. Instead of the light focusing on the retina, the light focuses in front of the retina. A myopic person can read a magazine; however the distance vision is blurry and requires glasses or contact lenses to make it clear.

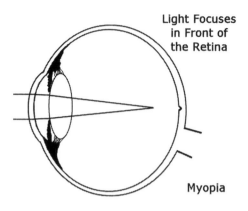

Figure 3   Myopia

Are More People Nearsighted Now Then in the Past?

It appears so. A study in the December 2009 issue of *Archives Of Ophthalmology* found a 66% increase in myopia when comparing the periods of 1971-1972 and 1999-2004.[1] This is a huge change over a thirty year period. The new study tried to simulate the testing methods of the original 1972 study on nearsightedness in the US population. The 1971-1972 National Health and Nutrition Examination Survey found that 25% of the US population between the ages of 12 and 54 were nearsighted vs. the 1994-2004 National Health and Nutrition Examination Survey's finding of 41.6%. Increased nearsightedness was noted regardless of age, sex, race, or education.

The authors concluded that it would be beneficial to identify behavioral risk factors that cause increased myopia. If risk factors for increasing myopia are identified, we may be able to slow the progression.

What Causes Nearsightedness?

As eye doctors, we are often asked what causes nearsightedness, and the usual answer is that we believe nearsightedness is a combination of genetics and environmental influences. In the last thirty years our society has become much more near centric. People spend hours glued to their computer monitors at work and home. Kids spend more time now than ever before with computer games, hand-held games, etc.

Finding ways to slow or halt the progression of myopia has been a longstanding subject of study in eyecare. The process of using special contact lenses to reshape the front part of a patient's eye to prevent the progression of nearsightedness and to allow the patient to see without glasses is called orthokeratology. For more information on preventing the progression of nearsightedness see page 181.

Farsightedness

What is Farsightedness?

Hyperopia, commonly referred to as farsightedness, occurs when a person has good distance vision but blurry near vision. Light entering the eye focuses behind the retina, placing a blurry image on the retina. For a hyperopic person to see clearly at any distance, a muscle inside the eye called the ciliary body, must focus an intra-ocular lens. As we get older, it becomes more difficult for the eye to accomplish this auto focusing. Because of the eye's ability to focus, farsighted people often don't need glasses until their thirties or forties. Uncorrected farsightedness, however, may cause a person to experience eyestrain or an eye turn (strabismus), depending on the degree of farsightedness and the patient's age. The younger we are, the easier it is for the eye to compensate for farsightedness. Uncorrected farsightedness can lead to amblyopia (for more information on amblyopia see page 166). Farsightedness is often confused with presbyopia.

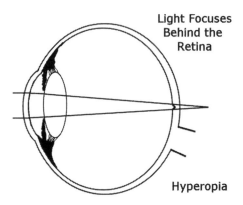

Light Focuses
Behind the
Retina

Hyperopia

Figure 4   Hyperopia; Farsightedness

Astigmatism

What is Astigmatism?

Many people feel astigmatism is a bad, progressive disease. Actually, astigmatism is caused when light focuses in two points in the back of the eye because the eye is not in the shape of a sphere. An eye with astigmatism has often been described as being in the shape of an egg or football. To some degree that is true, though an astigmatic eye is not exaggerated to that degree. Most people have some astigmatism. Visually, a person with uncorrected astigmatism will often see a faint shadow on letters or objects.

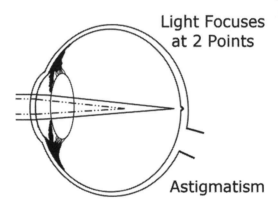

Figure 5   Astigmatism

How Do You Get Astigmatism?

Most people have some astigmatism. The amount of astigmatism, however, can change due to things such as trauma, scarring, corneal dystrophies, and intra-ocular lens dislocation.

Presbyopia

What Is Presbyopia?

As we mature, the crystalline lens of the eye loses its elasticity, thus reducing your ability to focus on near objects. You will notice this as your "arms get too short." This change is called presbyopia. This means you need a different correction for your close work than you need for your distance vision.

Presbyopia occurs as the eye's intra-ocular, crystalline lens loses its ability to focus light. The loss of focus results an inability to see at near, making reading glasses or bifocals necessary. A person can be both farsighted and presbyopic or nearsighted and presbyopic. Presbyopia typically begins in our early forties. The older we get the more difficult it is for our eyes to focus on objects that are near to us. The effects of presbyopia level off in our mid to late sixties.

Emmetropia

What Does Emmetropia Mean?

A person is emmetropic when an image focuses clearly on the retina without the aid of optical correction. A person who is emmetropic has uncorrected "normal vision."

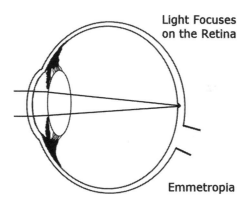

Figure 6   Emmetropia, Normal Vision

Dr. Richard A Driscoll

CHAPTER THREE

Lids And Lashes

We never think about this, but the eyelids and eyelashes are important in protecting our eyes. The eyelashes act as an early warning system, causing us to quickly and automatically blink at the first sign of a danger. The eyelids provide a degree of protection from not only physical danger, but they also serve to keep the eye moist allowing the eye to protect itself from infection and debris.

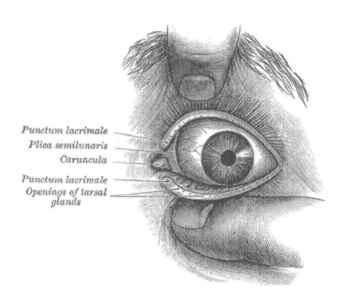

Punctum lacrimale
Plica semilunaris
Caruncula

Punctum lacrimale
Openings of tarsal glands

Figure 7   Eyelid Anatomy

Eyelid Conditions

Why Are My Eyelids Red And Itchy?

Blepharitis, meibomian gland dysfunction, and allergies are the leading causes of red, crusty, itchy eyes. All three are treated in a different manner, so an accurate diagnosis is important.

What Is Blepharitis?

Blepharitis is a common condition characterized by red, inflamed eyelids. Itching and flaking of the eyelids are also often associated with blepharitis.

What Causes Blepharitis?

Anterior blepharitis affects the outside front of the eyelid, where the eyelashes are attached. The two most common causes of anterior blepharitis are bacteria (usually Staphylococcus) and scalp dandruff.

Posterior blepharitis (also called meibomitis) affects the inner eyelid (the moist part that makes contact with the eye) and is caused by problems with the oil (meibomian) glands in this part of the eyelid. The meibomian glands become infected, usually by Staphylococcus bacteria. Two skin disorders can also cause this form of blepharitis: acne rosacea, which leads to red, inflamed skin, and scalp dandruff (seborrheic dermatitis).

What Are The Symptoms Of Blepharitis?

Symptoms of either form of blepharitis include a foreign body or burning sensation, excessive tearing, itching (usually at the lid margins), sensitivity to light (photophobia), red and swollen eyelids, redness of the eye, blurred vision, frothy tears, dry eye, or crusting of the eyelashes upon awakening.

What Other Conditions Are Associated With Blepharitis?

Styes (hordeolum), chalazions, acne rosacea, and dry eye syndrome are most often associated with blepharitis.

Abnormal or decreased oil secretions that are part of the tear film can result in excess tearing, or dry eye. Because tears are necessary to keep the cornea healthy, tear film problems can make people more at risk for corneal infections. For more information on dry eye syndrome see page 42.

If your eye doctor finds that acne rosacea is contributing to your blepharitis, we may also prescribe oral antibiotics in addition to the lid treatments.

Doc, This Thing On My Eye Hurts, What Is It?

Most often it is a hordeolum, more commonly known as a stye; a red tender bump on the eyelid caused by an acute infection of an oil (meibomian) gland.

A hordeolum exists in two forms, external and internal. An internal hordeolum is an infection deep within the tissue, a red painful lump. With time and/or treatment, an internal hordeolum usually becomes an external hordeolum. An external hordeolum becomes evident when you can see the white pussy stuff within the eyelid. This is called pointing. It is important to treat a stye early and aggressively. If left untreated, styes can turn into a chalazion.

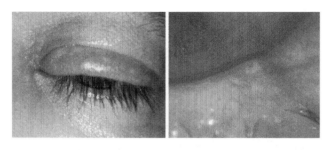

Figure 8   External (L) and Internal (R) Hordeolums

Do Those OTC Stye Medicines Work?

Generally, the over the counter stye medications are of limited benefit. A warm compress is a much more effective method of treating a stye. Seeing your eye doctor for oral or topical antibiotics will also shorten the course of the condition.

What Is This Painless Bump On My Eyelid?

Any bump on your eyelid should be checked out by your eye doctor. The most common painless bump is called a chalazion: This condition can follow the development of a stye. It is usually a painless firm lump caused by the leftover inflammatory products of a stye.

Styes are red, painful bumps on the eyelid that are often chronic problems for many patients. Styes are caused when the glands along the lid margin become clogged and infected, much like a pimple. Some patients are more susceptible to the recurrence of styes because they may have blepharitis, a common lid condition. If you should notice a small lump on your eyelid, it is best to see your eye doctor as soon as possible. The longer the treatment is delayed, the longer it will take to resolve it and the more painful it becomes. If a stye is not treated promptly or is large, a lump may remain. These lumps can be left alone or they may be removed surgically for aesthetic reasons.

How Is Blepharitis Treated?

Treatment for both forms of blepharitis involves keeping the lids clean and free of crusty exudate. Warm compresses should be applied to the lid to loosen the crusts, followed by a light scrubbing of the eyelid with a cotton swab and a mixture of water and baby shampoo. There are also some excellent commercially prepared lid scrubs that consist of a gauze-like pad soaked in a mild soap that you may find more convenient.

Because this is a chronic condition that rarely goes away completely, most patients must maintain an eyelid hygiene routine for life. You may notice significant improvement in three to five days; however, continue the treatment for the length of time prescribed by your eye doctor, (often one to two months with daily maintenance thereafter), otherwise your symptoms will likely return.

There are two forms of blepharitis, anterior blepharitis that involves the eyelashes, and posterior blepharitis that involves the meibomian glands behind the eyelashes.

What Is The Best Way To Do Lid Scrubs?

Soften eyelash crustiness with a very warm washcloth, placing it over your eyes for five minutes. There are three methods to performing lid scrubs.

Method A: Wrap a wet, warm washcloth around your finger. Dip washcloth in no-tears baby shampoo.

Method B: Dilute three drops of no-tears shampoo with one ounce of very warm water. Moisten a cotton tipped applicator with the mixture.

Method C: Use pre-moistened lid scrub preparation.

Scrub the lids at the base of the eyelashes. Scrub both the upper and lower lids.

Rinse the eyelids and face with warm, clear water.

Perform lid scrubs two to three times a day for one month. Once control is achieved, a maintenance schedule of once a day will usually keep the blepharitis in check. Often, your eye doctor will prescribe an antibiotic ointment or eye drops to use after you have done the lid scrubs. If an ointment is prescribed, place some on your finger or cotton-tipped applicator and smear it onto the base of both the upper and lower eyelashes. When the blepharitis is associated with scalp dandruff, a dandruff shampoo for the hair may also be prescribed.

How Should I Do Warm Compresses?

In the case of meibomitis, warm moist heat followed by massaging your lid margins will bring the disease under control. The following method is recommended.

Apply warm compresses to the lids for ten minutes

Fill a bowl with warm water from the hot water faucet (as hot as you can tolerate, without burning the skin).

Place a washcloth in the bowl and wring it out. Place the washcloth on the eye.

It is important to keep the temperature high during the ten minutes, therefore, repeat step two above every couple of minutes. You may find it helpful to have two washcloths, alternating with one on your eyes and one soaking.

Scrub the lids using the technique above for anterior blepharitis.

For posterior blepharitis or meibomitis, pressure should be applied to the upper and lower lid margins immediately following the warm compresses.

> If you have been diagnosed with a stye, do not apply pressure. Applying pressure will cause the stye to spread throughout the eyelid, making it worse. Skip the pressure step and proceed to rinsing your lid margins.

Trap the lid between your finger and the white part of your eye, making sure that the upper lid margin does not roll out. Apply pressure to the lid, squeezing the eyelid between your finger and the white part of the eye.

Repeat the above step all along the upper and lower lids. You may notice a milky white material extrude to the surface. This is what we want. The milky white "stuff" is the thick exudate within the meibomian gland coming to the surface. When the meibomian glands are plugged up with this thick exudate, it causes the lids to be red and swollen as well as exacerbating the dry eye symptoms.

Rinse the eyelids and face with warm, clear water.

Cosmetic Enhancement

I Want To Make My Eyelashes Longer Can You Tell Me About Latisse?

Latisse™ is currently the only FDA Approved medication to make your eyelashes longer, thicker, and darker. Latisse™ is a prescription medication that makes your own lashes longer, thicker, and fuller. Latisse™ contains 0.03% Bimatoprost, which is the same active ingredient as Allergan's glaucoma medication, Lumigan™. Doctors found that one of the side effects of Lumigan™ (as well as all medications of this type) was an increase in the darkness, thickness, length, and number of eyelashes. Lumigan™, a prescription eye medication not a cosmetic, grows impressive eyelashes in men and women alike.

Originally, Latisse™ was intended to be used in the treatment of hypotrichosis (the medical term for inadequate or insufficient eyelashes) in cancer patients who had lost their eyelashes while undergoing chemotherapy or radiation, but has now been approved by the FDA as an eyelash beautifier.

How Do I Know If Latisse™ Is Right For Me?

The first step is to schedule a consultation with your eye doctor where he or she will evaluate your medical history and examine you to determine if you are a good candidate for Latisse™.

Latisse™ is applied once a day, in the evening, to the base of the upper eyelashes with a single-use, sterile applicator. A new applicator is then used on the second eye. Repeating this daily will cause thicker, longer, darker, and more numerous eyelashes.

Allergan states that 4% of the patients experienced minor itching or eye redness. Latisse™ should not be used if you are allergic to the any of its components, have an active infection, or broken skin. Less common reactions are skin dryness, darkening or redness of the skin, or ocular irritation.

CHAPTER FOUR

Conjunctiva and Sclera

The sclera is the white part of the eye that gives the eye its rigidity, strength, and shape. The sclera is continuous with the cornea and is made primarily of irregularly layered collagen. The conjunctiva is the thin layer of transparent tissue extending from the corneal limbus, (where the colored part of the eye meets the white part) covering the sclera, and surrounding the rest of the eye. Small blood vessels are contained within the conjunctiva. The conjunctiva also covers the larger episcleral blood vessels. The conjunctiva contains many small glands responsible for keeping the eye moist by producing tears and mucous.

All About Pink Eyes, Yellow Eyes, And Red Eyes

I Think I Have Allergies. Do The OTC Allergy Medications Work?

April's showers not only bring May's flowers, but itchy, runny, and red eyes. With the increased rain, mold, and pollen levels increase dramatically, causing allergy sufferers to look like they were up all night.

Contact lens wearers seem to suffer most. It's hard to rub your eyes when you are wearing contacts. The good news is, there are many good allergy drops available, so you don't need to go without your contacts.

I would stay away from the over the counter drops such as Naphcon-A or Visine-A for allergies, etc. These drops contain medications that 15+ years ago were available by prescription only. In my experience, the old OTC allergy drops aren't as effective as the newer medications. Some of the newer OTC allergy drops, such as Zaditor, do bring relief for some patients. Today, however, many prescription medications do a much better job of controlling the redness and keeping our eyes from itching. Some of the current drops only need to be used once a day.

How Did I Get Pink Eye?

It depends. If a virus caused your pink eye, you probably infected yourself by touching something infected with the virus, then you touched your eye. For instance, someone with an active viral infection covers their mouth to cough or rubs their infected eye. You then shake hands with that person and rub your eye and, presto, in about a week your eye will look like you went on an all-night bender.

Almost always a viral eye infection is due to direct physical contact with something carrying the virus. Rarely will you contract a viral eye infection by being in the same room with someone (well, not unless they cough in your face). You get infected by handling something they handled. The best prevention is washing your hands.

Bacterial infections are spread the same way as a virus, by direct contact; however, viral eye infections are *much* more common as well as being more contagious.

Is Pink Eye Contagious?

Yes, a viral eye infection is quite contagious. Depending on the virus involved, an infected object can remain contaminated for hours. Don't share pillows, washcloths, etc with a person who has an eye infection. As a general rule, bacterial eye infections are less contagious.

What Is Pink Eye?

Pink eye is a descriptive term indicating that the eye is inflamed for some reason. Not all pink eyes are infected or contagious. "Pink" eye is usually caused by a virus (often quite contagious), allergies, or bacteria. The most common cause of pink eye is a viral infection or allergies. Patients with pink eye should not wear contact lenses. If you or your child have pink eye, it is best to see your eye doctor.

What Is This Yellow Spot On My Eye?

A pinguecula is the yellow bump on the white part of the eye, usually located at the 3:00 or 9:00 position. A pinguecula first starts out as a small white bump, with age, it usually turns yellow while increasing in size and height. When irritated, the pinguecula will become inflamed and turn a reddish color.

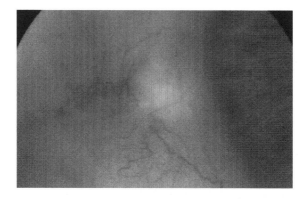

Figure 9   Pinguecula

I Want To Have This Yellow Thing On My Eye Removed

That yellow thing is probably a pinguecula. While it can be removed, the blood vessels that currently feed it may become larger after surgery, making your eye look worse. We almost always leave a pinguecula alone.

What Is This Huge Red Spot On My Eye?

If that big red spot is on the white part (sclera) of the eye and it seemed to appear rather suddenly, often overnight, then it may be a subconjunctival hemorrhage.

The white part of the eye is covered with layers of clear tissue. The layer closes to the sclera is called the episcleral and the next layer is called the called the conjunctiva. Within and below the conjunctiva are numerous, small blood vessels. When one of these blood vessels springs a leak (some of the most common reasons are listed in the next question) the blood will pool between these clear. It does not take much blood, typically only a few drops, to spread out, and make the eye look very red.

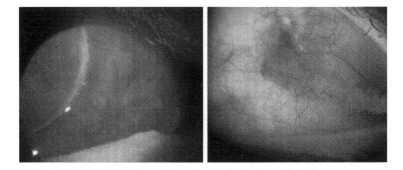

Figure 10   Subconjunctival Hemorrhage

What Causes A Subconjunctival Hemorrhage?

Subconjunctival hemorrhages can be caused by many different factors, for this reason, it is recommended that you be seen by your eye doctor. It is not always possible to determine the cause of all subconjunctival hemorrhages, however the most common causes, in no particular order, are;

- Trauma, surgical and physical
- Infection, bacterial and viral
- Medications
- High blood pressure
- Genetic blood disorders

My Doctor Says I Have A Subconjunctival Hemorrhage, How Long Will My Eye Be Red?

Subconjunctival hemorrhages are a lot like bruises, however instead of the blood being trapped between muscle fibers, the blood is trapped between clear layers of tissue. The blood will be resorbed by your body, typically resolving completely in seven to fourteen days. Your eye may look worse before looking better as the blood spreads out before being resorbed. The red color will probably transition for red, to yellow, to white.

Dr. Richard A Driscoll

CHAPTER FIVE

The Cornea

The cornea is the clear surface at the front of the eye. The cornea operates as a fixed focus lens and is the primary refractive surface of the eye. Quite strong and thin, the average cornea is slightly over .5 mm thick (500 microns is approximately .2 inches). The cornea is made primarily of collagen fibers. The cornea is made up of five layers, the epithelium, Bowman's layer, the stroma, Descemet's membrane, and the endothelium.

What Is The White Ring Around My Eye?

Corneal arcus is an opacification of the cornea appearing as a white ring inside the white part (sclera) of the eye and over the iris. As we age we are more likely to have corneal arcus, however corneal arcus in a young person, that would be a person under 40 . . . ahem, has been tied to elevated cholesterol levels. The presence of corneal arcus in patients under 40 does not mean they have high cholesterol, however; their odds of having elevated cholesterol levels are higher thus a lipid panel is recommended.

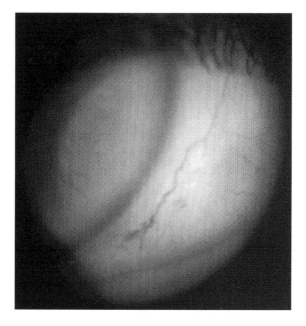

Figure 11   Corneal Arcus

Dry Eye Syndrome

Dry eye related discomfort is one of the most frequent complaints heard by eye doctors. The symptoms of dry eyes are varied, and the list below is by no means all-inclusive; however, patients who suffer from dry eyes usually experience a number of the symptoms.

What are the Symptoms of Dry Eye Syndrome?

- dryness
- burning sensation
- excess watering/tearing
- redness
- stinging sensation
- a foreign body sensation
- scratchiness
- light sensitivity
- sandy/gritty sensation
- blurred vision
- excess mucous
- contact lens intolerance

What Causes Dry Eye Syndrome?

Dry eye syndrome, often referred to as keratitis sicca or keratoconjunctivitis sicca, is caused by insufficient and/or poor quality tears.

There are three main components to human tears. The bulk of human tears are produced by the lacrimal gland. This oily component of the tears is produced by the meibomian glands and is responsible for keeping the tears from evaporating too quickly. The third component, the goblet cells, keeps all of the other components mixed as an emulsion. When one of the parts of this mixture becomes unbalanced, patients become symptomatic. There are numerous reasons as to why these glands may not be doing their part.

Insufficient tear production and/or poor tear quality are the most common causes of dry eye syndrome. Inflammation of the lacrimal gland is the most common cause of insufficient tear volume. Meibomian gland dysfunction, inflammation of the glands at the eyelid margin, contributes to poor tear quality. Medications frequently cause ocular dryness. The medications most commonly causing dry eyes are antihistamines, oral contraceptives, and decongestants and diuretics. Hormonal changes also contribute to insufficient and poor quality tears.

Why Are My Eyes So Dry Lately?

Many conditions can contribute to dry eyes, including both your health and your environment. Are you near any ceiling fans or heaters? Does your car's heater or air conditioner blow directly on your eyes? Some medications, such as antihistamines, decongestants, and diuretics can also contribute to dryness. Hormonal changes, such as those attributed to pregnancy or menopause, may also be a factor. Some people have a condition called blepharitis, where their lids become dry and flaky. This, too, can contribute to dryness. Systemic conditions, such as Sjögren's Syndrome, an autoimmune disorder where the glands of the mucous membrane are attacked, can also be contributing factors to dry eye syndrome.

Your eye doctor can evaluate the source of your dry eyes and initiate a treatment plan. Dry eye syndrome is common and can be successfully treated. In addition to eye drops there are many new solutions for the treatment of dry eyes that don't require the use of eye drops.

Who Is At Risk For Dry Eye Syndrome?

Dry eye syndrome is common. It is estimated that between 10% and 30% of the general population experiences dry eyes, resulting in up to ninety million affected individuals in the United States.[2] The incidence of dry eye syndrome is higher, however, in those over age forty and in women.[3,4,5]

What Are The Most Common Causes Of Dry Eye Syndrome?

Dry eye syndrome is usually caused by a number of factors and, as such its treatment usually involves multiple components. The most common causes of dry eye syndrome are systemic causes, refractive surgery, contact lenses, and medications.

What Are The Systemic Causes of Dry Eye Syndrome?

Some systemic disorders such as Sjögren syndrome, rheumatoid arthritis, and acne rosacea make a person more likely to experience ocular dryness.

Why Does Refractive Surgery Make My Eyes Dry?

Refractive surgery procedures such as PRK, LASIK, and LASEK disrupt the neural feedback loop and are common causes of dry eyes. Poor quality and insufficient tears can cause both decreased visual acuity and discomfort for refractive surgery patients and needs to be addressed during all phases of a refractive surgery patient's care.

Can Contact Lenses Cause Dry Eye Syndrome?

Patients often report that their eyes do not seem to be dry until they wear contact lenses. Contact lenses don't cause the dryness; however, a patient with dry eyes will experience discomfort because their eyes cannot support the presence of the contact lens. Typically, soft contact lenses are 30 to 70% water. Contact lenses essentially work like a sponge in the eye. A patient with borderline dry eye symptoms is often contact lens intolerant. Contact lenses rely on our eyes to produce enough tears to hydrate the contact lenses, allowing them to float on a cushion of tears. If there are not enough tears to both hydrate the contact lens and lubricate the eye, the patient experiences discomfort often leading to contact lens intolerance. Often a contact lens intolerant patient can wear contact lenses for a few hours, but the wearing time decreases when in the presence of smoke, air conditioning, wind, and low humidity.

Don't necessarily give up on wearing contact lenses if you find them uncomfortable. Seek a consult for dry eyes with your eye doctor. Most patients find that by treating the dry eye symptoms, they can greatly improve their contact lens comfort and wearing time.

Can Medications Make My Eyes Dry?

Numerous medications will contribute to dry eye syndrome. The most common culprits are antihistamines, decongestants, birth control pills, diuretics, and anti-acne medications.

How Is Dry Eye Syndrome Diagnosed?

Dry eye syndrome is diagnosed in the office by considering the clinical presentation, patient's complaints and diagnostic testing. Determining the cause of the dryness whether it is insufficient tear production, poor tear quality or a systemic disease is critical in improving your comfort.

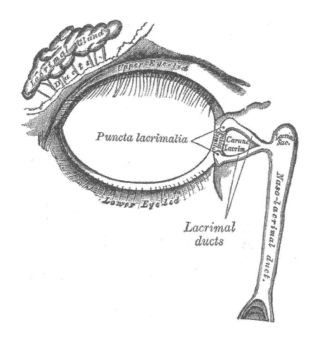

Figure 12   The Lacrimal (Tear) System

How Is Dry Eye Syndrome Treated?

Treatment is often accomplished through numerous different courses of action. Artificial tears containing active ingredients such as carboxymethylcellulose and polyvinyl alcohol are helpful in mild cases of dry eye syndrome. Moderate to severe cases are often treated with a combination of artificial tears, punctal occlusion, and medications such as ophthalmic steroids and Restasis®.

There are numerous treatments available to patients with dry eyes. The treatment, of course, depends on the cause of the dryness. Systemic causes of ocular dryness, such as acne rosacea, medications, and endocrine imbalance must be addressed first. If symptoms persist, other treatments are initiated, such as artificial tears, the use of medications that promote tearing such as Restasis®, and punctal plugs to prevent the tears that are produced from being drained into the nose. Increasing the Omega-3 fatty acids in one's diet can also reduce dry eye symptoms significantly.

Address Underlying Conditions

The first course of action is to address any underlying factors contributing to the symptoms such as the systemic, causes mentioned earlier. Infections of the eyelids, such as blepharitis and meibomitis, must also be treated before any other treatment is initiated. Often treatment of the underlying conditions still leaves patients symptomatic, and additional treatment is required to provide adequate relief.

Artificial Tears

Artificial tears containing active ingredients such as carboxymethylcellulose, hydroxypropyl methylcellulose, glycerin, castor oil, polyethyline glycol, or polyvinyl alcohol are used in mild cases of dry eyes. Not all artificial tear brands work the same or work for all patients. More severe cases of dry eye syndrome require additional treatment. If you find yourself using your artificial tears three or more times a day, you should use a preservative-free tear. Most patients find that artificial tears do help; however, the affect is only temporary, lasting only ten to fifteen minutes. Most of these patients will experience significant relief with punctal occlusion.

Punctal Occlusion

In my clinical experience, significant dry eye relief is achieved with punctal occlusion. The puncta is the small opening found on the edge of the upper and lower eyelids next to the nose. Tears drain out of the eye through the puncta into the nose. This is why your nose runs when you cry. If you aren't producing enough tears, you don't want the tears that you are producing to be drained away. Punctal occlusion is painless and performed in the office, taking only a couple of minutes.

If your dry eyes are not responding to artificial tears and ointments, your eye doctor can insert temporary collagen plugs into the tiny openings of the ducts that drain your tears. With these plugs in place, your tears and any artificial tears you may add will stay in contact with your eyes for a much longer period of time, relieving your symptoms. This process is totally painless and takes only a few minutes. These temporary plugs dissolve in five to seven days and, if successful, can be replaced with non-dissolvable silicone plugs that can be removed at a later date if needed.

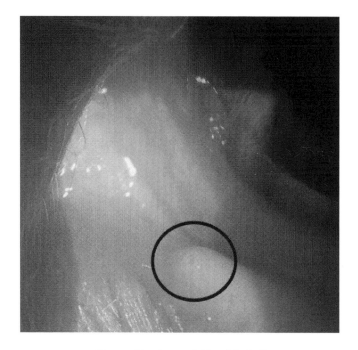

Figure 13   Punctal Plug (circled)

Dietary Changes

Numerous studies have shown that increasing our dietary intake of Omega-3 fatty acids, such as those found in oily fish like salmon, are beneficial. Western diets almost never contain enough Omega-3 fatty acids to provide a therapeutic benefit; therefore, dietary supplementation is almost always required. For more information on Omega-3 fatty acids see page 61.

Medications

Pharmaceutical manufacturers have focused a significant portion of their considerable resources into dry eye medications. Restasis® is the first of many medications being developed for dry eye patients. We have found Restasis® to be helpful in patients when the underlying cause of their symptoms is insufficient tear volume due to inflammation of the lacrimal gland. Restasis® does not provide immediate relief; a therapeutic benefit is usually noted in two to four months.

In patients with severe dry eyes a mild ophthalmic steroid may provide added benefit. Currently, there is a lot of research being done to find medications that effectively treat dry eye syndrome. I expect within the next five years we will have numerous additional medications to add to our dry eye treatment regimen.

Contact Lens Changes

Merely changing the type of contact lens is rarely enough to provide sufficient, consistent relief; however, careful selection of the contact lens material may often be beneficial and is one of the many treatment options available. See page 69 for more information on contact lens options.

Conjunctival Inserts

LACRISERT® is available for the treatment of dry eye syndrome. In our experience, the results have been mixed. LACRISERT® is inserted inside your lower lid once or twice a day. The LACRISERT® slowly releases supplemental tears to your eyes throughout the day.

Most patients have found that using the LACRISERT® once a day provides sufficient relief for most of the workday. When the LACRISERT® has almost completely dissolved, it tends not to stay trapped inside the lower lid, causing intermittent blurred vision. A drop of artificial tears flushes out the last remnant, restoring vision.

There is no silver bullet to dry eye treatment; however, management almost always results in significant improvement in comfort. Symptomatic relief usually involves a multifaceted, systematic approach.

Overview of Keratoconus

Keratoconus (ker-uh-toe-KOH-nus) is one of the most common corneal dystrophies in the U.S., affecting approximately one in every 2000 Americans.[6] It is usually first diagnosed in teenagers and adults in their twenties.

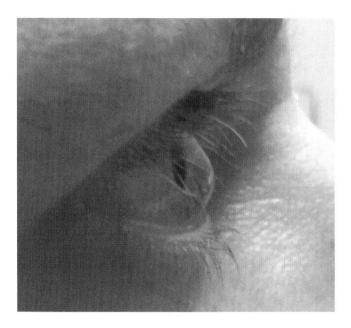

Figure 14   Profile View Of A Patient With Keratoconus

What is Keratoconus?

Keratoconus is a progressive thinning of the cornea. The cornea is the clear, front window of the eye, which, along with the intraocular lens, focuses light onto the retina. The cornea normally is a smooth, round, dome-like shape; however, in keratoconus, the cornea becomes thin, irregular, and starts to protrude from the center or just below the center like a cone. This causes blurry vision that is often not fully correctable with glasses. Keratoconus usually involves both eyes; however, one eye may be more advanced than the other. Below is the corneal topography of a patient with early keratoconus.

Notice the darkened, round areas near the center in the photos below. That is the "cone" that protrudes from the cornea. For an example of a normal corneal topography, see the figure on page 90.

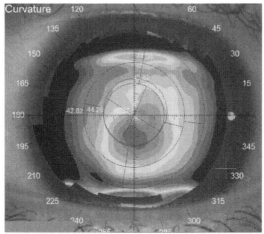

Early Keratoconus Topography

Figure 15   Mild Keratoconus

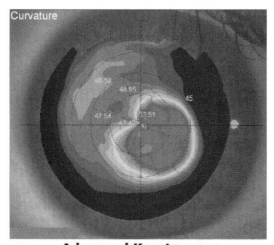

Advanced Keratoconus

Figure 16   Corneal Topography, Advanced Keratoconus

What are the Symptoms Of Keratoconus?

Typically blurred vision that cannot be corrected with eyeglasses is the first symptom of keratoconus.

What Causes Keratoconus?

Studies indicate that keratoconus stems from several possible causes:

1. An inherited corneal abnormality. About eight percent of those with the condition have a family history of keratoconus.

2. An eye injury, i.e., excessive eye rubbing.

3. Keratoconus has been associated with certain eye diseases, such as retinitis pigmentosa, retinopathy of prematurity, and vernal keratoconjunctivitis.

4. Systemic conditions such as Leber's congenital amaurosis, Ehlers-Danlos Syndrome, Marfan's Syndrome, Down's Syndrome, and osteogenesis imperfecta have been associated with keratoconus.

How Is Keratoconus Treated?

Contact lenses are the treatment of choice for keratoconus. Over 90% of patients with keratoconus will be successfully treated with contact lenses. In the early stages of keratoconus your vision can often be corrected with eyeglasses or standard contact lenses: however, as the corneal thinning worsens, we must rely on specially fitted contact lenses to reduce the distortion and provide better visual acuity. Cross Linking, though not a cure and not yet FDA approved, shows great promise in improving the vision of keratoconus patients. Approximately 10% of keratoconus patients will not achieve satisfactory vision with contacts or glasses and will have a corneal transplant.

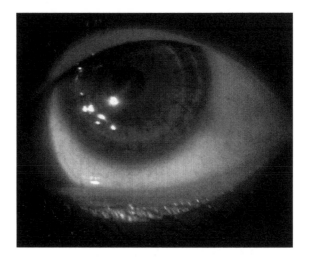

Figure 17   Corneal Transplant, 2 Weeks Post Op

How Are Contact Lenses Used To Treat Keratoconus?

The contact lens fitting process involves making a computerized topographical map of your cornea. A topographical map allows your doctor to see the exact size and position of your "cone." By using corneal topography, a lens can be designed that will provide much better vision and comfort than traditional contact lenses.

Typically, your eye doctor will use the topographical data to select an initial diagnostic lens from a set of standardized keratoconus lenses. The contact lens will be placed on your eye. Once the lens has stabilized on the eye, the fit and vision are evaluated. Multiple diagnostic lenses may be necessary to aid your doctor in designing a contact lens just for you.

When you receive your initial customized contact lens, your doctor will evaluate how the special curves on the back surface of the lens match the curves of your eye. Often it is necessary to modify the way the initial lens fits on your eye; therefore, it is normal for it to take numerous office visits and lens adjustments to arrive at a lens that gives you good visual acuity along with a good physiological fit and comfort.

Patients with keratoconus have more sensitive corneas, and some awareness of the lens is not uncommon during the early fitting of the lens. First time lens wearers may require an adaptation period before good comfort is attained.

What New Contact Lens Treatment Options Are Available?

Recently, a few new types of keratoconic lenses have come available. The first brings together the visual acuity of a gas permeable lens and the comfort of a soft lens. This lens is called the SynergEyes lens. It uses a small gas permeable lens surrounded by a soft lens skirt. Synergeyes lenses can actually be used for any contact lens patient; however, we have found it to be especially helpful not only for patients with keratoconus, but also irregular astigmatism, pellucid marginal degeneration, and patients who have had complications due to RK, LASIK or PRK.

Mini scleral lenses are another relatively new option for keratoconic patients as well as patients with irregular corneas from refractive surgery or corneal transplant. A mini scleral lens is about the size of a small, soft contact lens, thus making it a comfortable lens to wear. Patients often state it is almost as comfortable as a soft lens. This increased comfort over traditional gas permeable lenses is due to its size. The upper edge of a mini scleral lens sits under the upper eyelid, giving much better comfort when a patient blinks.

When Is A Corneal Transplant Needed?

In most cases, the cornea will stabilize after a few years. The vast majority of patients with keratoconus are best treated with the new hybrid contact lenses or gas permeable contact lenses. In about 10% of patients with keratoconus, the cornea will eventually become too scarred to achieve good vision, will not tolerate a contact lens, or repeated episodes of acute corneal hydrops will result in a corneal transplant being necessary

A corneal transplant or penetrating keratoplasty is successful in approximately 90% of those with advanced keratoconus. Several studies have also reported that 74% or more of these patients have 20/40 vision or better after the operation.[7] In most cases contact lenses or glasses will still be necessary to achieve the best visual acuity following a corneal transplant. Nearly 90% of keratoconus patient's corneal grafts remained viable after ten years and 49% after twenty years. Therefore, young patients receiving a corneal graft may expect to have more than one during their lifetime.

What Is Corneal Collagen Cross Linking?

Corneal collagen cross linking (CXL) is the newest development in the treatment of keratoconus and, as such, it holds a lot of promise. Quite simply, CXL involves treating the cornea with riboflavin, then activating its collagen cross linking properties with ultraviolet light. The increased cross linking not only increases the strength of the cornea, but usually flattens the cornea as well. Currently, CXL is available on an experimental basis in the United States as it goes through the FDA approval process. While CXL appears to stabilize and somewhat flatten the cornea, patients still may require contact lenses or glasses to achieve their best visual acuity.

How Are Intracorneal Rings Used To Treat Keratoconus?

Intacs are translucent, plastic semi-circles originally developed as an alternative method of treating myopia, an alternative to LASIK. Intacs are now FDA approved to treat keratoconus as well as 1.00 to 3.00 diopters of myopia. A small incision is made into the cornea, and the Intac is then inserted within the cornea on either side of the cone. Think of it as inserting a tube under the ground next to a mountain in an attempt to raise the ground around the mountain, thus lowering the mountain's relative height with its surroundings.

I Have Keratoconus Why Does My Eye Hurt?

The hallmark of acute pain in keratoconus patients is an episode of acute corneal hydrops. Light sensitivity and a decrease in vision are also often associated with corneal hydrops. Most cases of acute corneal hydrops will get better with time, and seeing your keratoconus specialist during an episode can ease the process greatly. Corneal scarring following an episode of hydrops may make the cornea stronger; however, the scars may interfere with vision. Repeated episodes of corneal hydrops will often cause a patient to seek a corneal transplant

What Research Is Being Done About Keratoconus?

The National Eye Institute is conducting a natural history study called the Collaborative Longitudinal Evaluation of Keratoconus Study (CLEK) to identify factors that influence the severity and progression of keratoconus. The CLEK Study closed enrollment in June 1996 with over 1200 patients and ended in 2004. The CLEK study spawned over 35 papers. If you need some good night time reading, you can find a list of them here http://bit.ly/CLEKPapers or http://bit.ly/CLEKPapers2

What Can I Do To Prevent My Keratoconus From Getting Worse?

The single most important thing for you to do is to have your keratoconus specialist evaluate the physiological fit of your contact lenses and your corneal health every six to twelve months. A poorly fitting contact lens may cause additional scarring; therefore, it is best to have your corneal health and contact lenses evaluated regularly.

Having a current pair of glasses as a backup to your contact lenses is also important. You will probably see better with your contacts than your glasses; however, there are times when your eyes need a break, and having a pair of glasses that you don't actually mind being seen wearing will make you more likely to give your eyes that occasional, much needed break.

What Can I Expect Over The Coming Years?

For the vast majority of patients the fact that they have keratoconus will not negatively affect their daily life. Having keratoconus means you will need regular eye care, as discussed above. It also means that the best vision you can attain with your glasses will likely not be as good as that vision you achieve with your contact lenses. Over the years your vision will fluctuate just like everyone else's.

Pterygium

What Is This Pink Fleshy Thing Growing Over My Eye?

A pterygium (pronounced ter-ij-ee-um) is the fleshy growth usually located at the 3:00 or 9:00 position that grows over the colored part of the eye.

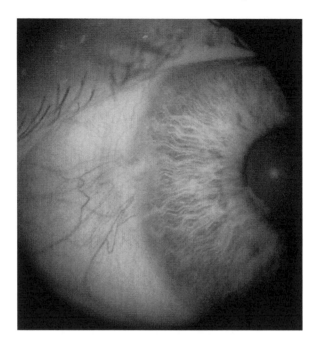

Figure 18   Pterygium

What Causes A Pterygium?

Ultraviolet light and ocular irritation are the most common causes. A pterygium is most commonly found in people who spend a lot of time outdoors. People who spent their youth within twenty degrees of the equator are more likely to develop a pterygium.

Dr. Richard A Driscoll

CHAPTER SIX

Nutritional Supplements

Nutritional supplements have become an increasingly important part of a physician's treatment plan in all medical specialties. Eye care is no different. The most common use of nutritional supplements in eye care is in the treatment of dry eye syndrome and macular degeneration.

Fish Oil and Omega-3 Fatty Acids

Our Western diets are low in fish, thus we often don't get enough of the Omega-3 fatty acids; therefore, supplementation is quite common. Our grocery stores, health food stores, and pharmacies offer a plethora of choices. Most questions center around do Omega-3 fatty acids work and how do I find the right one.

Doc, What Is All This I Hear About Fish Oil Capsules and Omega-3s?

Omega-3 fatty acids, also known as essential fatty acids, are an important component in our treatment of dry eye syndrome and macular degeneration, not to mention the added and well documented benefit that Omega-3 fatty acids provide in Alzheimer's Disease and cholesterol.

Are All Fish Oil Capsules Created Equal?

How to Select the Best Source of Omega-3 Fatty Acids

As eye doctors, we often recommend that our patients with dry eyes increase their dietary intake of Omega-3 fatty acids. When questioned, I find that a surprising number of patients are already taking fish oil capsules; however, they are almost never taking enough. Our typical dosage is 2000 mg to 3000 mg in a combination of eicosapentaenoic acid (EPA) and docosahexaenoic acid (DHA). This translates into approximately 4 oz of wild, Atlantic salmon per day. Regardless of how much we like salmon, we probably don't want it every day no matter how many different ways there are to fix it; therefore, fish oil capsules are a necessary dietary supplement. Mercury consumption can also be a consideration, especially in the case of farmed salmon.

Generally, oily fish such as salmon, anchovy, mackerel and herring are high in Omega-3 fatty acids. It is easy to recommend that we increase the Omega-3 fatty acids in our diet due to their many well documented health benefits in conditions such as dry eye syndrome,[8] macular degeneration, Alzheimer's disease, and lowering triglyceride and cholesterol levels.

A high quality fish oil capsule should have the following qualities

1. High in the Omega-3 essential fatty acids eicosapentaenoic acid (EPA) and docosahexaenoic acid (DHA)

2. Be of a concentrated form (which also removes heavy metals such as mercury)

3. The Omega-3 fatty acids should be in the triglyceride form and not the ester form

4. Should not taste like fish

Always read the label and look for the amount of EPA and DHA. There may also be some other Omega-3 fatty acids in the capsule; however, EPA will make up the bulk of the Omega-3s. At least 50%

of the capsule's contents/weight should be of the Omega-3 fatty acids.

Am I Using Concentrated Omega-3 Fatty Acids?

If the Omega-3 content of the capsule is less than 50%, this is not a concentrated Omega-3 capsule and you should find another. One of the reasons why you want to only purchase concentrated Omega-3 capsules is so that any mercury has been removed. Also if the capsule uses concentrated Omega-3s, it is unlikely you will experience indigestion and "fish burp." If you use the non concentrated fish oil capsules, you will need to consume eight or more capsules to attain a therapeutic level of EPA and DHA. Consuming eight or more non-concentrated fish oil capsules will virtually ensure digestive problems, ultimately leading to a discontinuation of the treatment. Furthermore, you should avoid Omega-3 capsules with an enteric coating. A high quality fish oil capsule should not need a "special coating" to make it easier to tolerate.

Which Is Better The Triglyceride Form or Ester Form of Fish Oil?

The triglyceride form of the Omega-3 fatty acids is the same form as that found in fish. A fish oil capsule manufacturer may elect to leave the fish oil in the ester form because it is cheaper. During the concentration process, the fish oil is converted into the ester form where the fish oil is concentrated, purified, and the fish taste is removed. The fish oil must then be converted back into the triglyceride form. The triglyceride form is more bio-efficient; our bodies can more readily utilize the triglyceride form of these essential fatty acids.

Which Is A Better Source Of Omega-3 Fatty Acids, Fish Oil Or Flax Seed Meal?

Flax is commonly recommended as a source high in Omega-3 fatty acids. However, is it an efficient source of bio-available Omega-3 fatty acids?

The short answer, without question, is fish oil. We have found better results treating dry eye syndrome by eliminating the flax seed oil and greatly increasing the EPA and DHA. As stated previously, we recommend 2000 mg to 3000 mg of EPA and DHA combined. Flax seed oil is unstable, thus has a short shelf life at room temperature. Flax seed oil also does not contain Omega-3 fatty acids. Instead, our bodies must convert the ALA (alpha linolenic acid) contained within the flax seed into the Omega-3 fatty acids that can then be used by our bodies. Another disadvantage to flax seed oil is that our body's conversion of flax seed oil to EPA or DHA is very inefficient.

The conversion rate of ALA to EPA/DHA has been reported to be between 4% and 15% (worse for DHA than EPA and lower for men than women). A person's conversion rate can vary based on many factors. Therefore, fish is a much better, more efficient source of Omega-3 fatty acids.

Can I Use Flax Seed Meal In The Treatment Of Dry Eye Syndrome?

For strict dietary vegans, flax may be the only option of increasing the Omega-3 fatty acids, albeit an inefficient one. However, for most people, flax seed oil's role is limited in the treatment of dry eye syndrome. Flax seed meal, on the other hand, may have a limited role.

The biggest disadvantages to using flax seed oil is that you can't cook with it (it is not stable above 160° F), it must be refrigerated, and it has a short shelf life. Flax seed meal, on the other, hand can be used as a shortening substitute, has a high fiber content, has a much longer shelf life, and can be used in baking. Therefore, I would only recommend flax seed oil if someone did not like the texture of the flax seed meal, or flax meal would be inappropriate in a particular recipe. One of flax seed meal's greatest advantages is its high fiber content. Therefore, I would recommend flax seed meal in baking to increase our dietary fiber, and any ALA converted to the omega fatty acids is just an extra bonus.

In addition, flax seeds are not digested by our bodies and should not be considered as a dietary source of fiber or Omega-3 fatty acids. The flax seed's shell is hard and must be crushed if our bodies are to utilize it. Therefore, flax meal is a better source of Omega-3 fatty acids than flax seeds.

What About Krill Oil As A Source Of Omega-3 Fatty Acids?

Krill oil can be an acceptable source of Omega-3 fatty acids; however, just like with fish oil, read the label and see how much EPA and DHA are actually contained in the krill oil capsule. In my experience krill, oil is not a cost effective source of Omega-3 fatty acids.

Omega-3 Essential Fatty Acids Recommendations

It is hard to beat fish oil derived from the oily fish such as mackerel, salmon, and anchovy as a safe, cost effective source of Omega-3 fatty acids. Always read the label to determine how much EPA and DHA is contained within the capsule you are taking. Purchase fish oil capsules, in the triglyceride form, that have had the mercury and other heavy metals removed. The typical dosage should be 2000 mg to 3000 mg, of a combination of EPA and DHA, per day.

Nutritional Supplements For Macular Degeneration

What Can I Do To Prevent Macular Degeneration?

The short answer is greatly increasing the antioxidants in our diet, stop smoking, seek regular eye exams at the interval recommend by your doctor, and monitor your vision with an Amsler Grid (for more specific recommendations on macular degeneration see page 127).

Is There A Link Between Smoking And AMD?

That would be a resounding YES (I'll bet you can hear me all the way from Texas, right?). As if there aren't enough reasons to stop smoking already, if you are a smoker, stopping smoking is probably the single best thing you can do to prevent macular degeneration. Smokers have a four times greater risk of getting macular degeneration than non-smokers.[9]

What Is The AREDS Study?

The Age Related Eye Disease Study 1 (AREDS1) was a long-term study where 3640 patients were followed for an average of 6 ½ years to see if antioxidant nutritional supplements affected the progression of macular degeneration or cataracts. AREDS1 showed that the supplements had no affect on cataracts;[10] however, in regard to age-related macular degeneration (AMD), it showed that the number of patients progressing from moderate AMD to severe AMD was reduced by 25%.[11] The data collected from the AREDS1 is still producing publications giving us a much better understanding of macular degeneration

The initial AREDS1 study provided many answers; however, as with most studies of this scale, it raised questions resulting in another study. AREDS2 is studying the affect of lutein, zeazanthin, and/or

Omega-3 fatty acids on cataracts and macular degeneration. AREDS2 will also evaluate the effect of eliminating beta-carotene and/or zinc from the supplement formula on the progression of AMD. AREDS2 is currently ongoing, with the conclusion expected to be in 2013 or 2014.

What Is In The AREDS 1 and 2 Formulas?

The AREDS1 Formula

- Vitamin C 500 mg

- Vitamin E 400 IU

- Beta-carotene 15 mg

- Zinc Oxide 80 mg

- Cupric Oxide 2mg

The AREDS2 formula

- Lutein 10 mg

- Zeaxanthin 2 mg

- DHA 350 mg

- EPA 650 mg

Do The Omega-3s Help With Macular Degeneration?

Yes, numerous studies have shown that the Omega-3 essential fatty acids have a positive affect on reducing the progression of macular degeneration. AREDS2 is the first large scale study (over 3000 patients), long-term study to evaluate the effect of Omega-3 fatty acids on AMD. The Blue Mountain Eye Study found that patients who consumed at least one serving of fish per week and had low Omega-6 fatty acid consumption experienced some protection from early AMD. Incidentally, the same study also found that tree nuts had a similar affect on AMD.[12] Another study found that female health professionals who had not been diagnosed with AMD were less likely to later be diagnosed with AMD if they consumed one or more servings of fish per week.[13] It has also been shown that the genetic risk of developing early AMD can be greatly reduced (by about 1/3) by taking DHA/EPA and antioxidants such as zinc, zeaxanthin, and lutein.[14]

CHAPTER SEVEN

Contact Lenses

Perhaps you are a contact lens wearer. Do you remember the first time you put your contacts in? Do you remember commenting how the trees have thousands of individual leaves instead of one big, green mass? I remember being amazed at how nice it was to see without those eyeglass frames getting in the way, without my lenses steaming up when I came in from the outside. It was great. Ahh, the freedom of contact lenses.

Contact lenses have come a long way since I first started wearing them in the early eighties. They are more comfortable, easier to care for (remember plugging them into the wall to "cook" them?), healthier for the eyes, less expensive, with much wider range of options. Contact lenses have a lot to offer and, with that, many questions. I hope you find what you are looking for.

Contact Lens Options

What Are Gas Permeable Contact Lenses?

The precursor to the modern gas permeable contact lens was the hard lens. Hard lenses were made of polymethylmethacrylate (PMMA) more commonly known as Plexiglas. Hard lenses gave patients excellent vision; however, they were impermeable to oxygen resulting blurry vision with glasses following removal of the lenses.

The introduction of gas permeable lenses allowed for significant improvements in lens design, resulting in more comfortable lenses, and minimal blur with glasses after removal. Some gas permeable lenses are approved for overnight wear.

What Are Soft Contact Lenses?

Soft contact lenses are made out of a pliable material that feels like the plastic wrap used to cover food. Hydrophilic materials are used to make soft contact lenses; therefore, water accounts for up to 70% of a soft contact's weight.

What Are Spherical Contacts?

Spherical contact lenses are used to correct myopia or hyperopia without astigmatism. The most common type of contact lenses are spherical lenses. Gas permeable and soft contact lenses are available as spherical contacts.

What Are Toric Contact lenses?

Patients with astigmatism usually require toric contact lenses to achieve sharp vision. Toric contacts have two curves to correct the astigmatism and are often thicker at the bottom. The increased thickness allows the lenses to remain in the same position, providing stable vision, at all times. Both gas permeable and soft contact lenses are available in toric contact lens designs. For more information about astigmatism see page 23.

How Long Are Contact Lenses Worn?

Contact lenses are usually removed before going to bed; however, some contact lenses have been approved by the FDA for extended wear, allowing patients to sleep while the lenses remain in their eyes. Some contact lenses have been approved for occasional overnight wear (called flexible wear), usually once or twice a week, but not multiple, consecutive nights. More common however, are contact lenses approved for up to 6 nights of continuous wear followed by a night without the lenses. A couple of contacts are approved for up to 30 nights of continuous wear.

Keep in mind that these are only recommendations for the maximum number of nights to sleep in your lenses. Just because a lens is approved for extended wear doesn't mean you have to take advantage of that option. Many patients, and doctors alike, prefer extended wear contact lenses because they allow more air to get to the eye than traditional lenses; however, patients continue to remove the lenses nightly.

What Soft Contact Lens Replacement Options Are Available?

When soft contact lenses were first introduced in the early 1970s patients wore the same pair of lenses for an entire year. Soon doctors began to spend a significant amount of time resolving the complications that occurred with wearing the same pair of contacts for such long periods. Almost forty years later, doctors rarely prescribe annual replacement contact lenses. Contact lenses are now available with daily, bi-weekly, monthly and quarterly replacement options.

What Are Daily Replacement Contacts?

Daily replacement is the fastest growing contact lens modality in the United States. In Europe and Japan, daily replacement contacts are already the most popular option. Daily contacts offer the ultimate in convenience, you are always wearing a new, fresh lens. Contact lens deposits are never a problem which is especially helpful for patients with dry eyes. Cleaning of daily lenses is not necessary. They are extremely convenient for travel. Daily contact lenses offer the lowest rate of contact lens related problems.

What Are Bi-weekly (2-week) Replacement Contacts?

Two week contact lenses are the most commonly prescribed contacts lenses in the United States. Patients are usually asked to replace their contact lenses on the 1st and 15th of the month. Two week contact lenses still require daily cleaning and disinfection, however; the use of enzyme tablets is no longer recommended. Patients wearing the two week contact lenses tend to have the lowest compliance rate with replacing their lenses as prescribed. Monthly lenses seem to have a higher replacement compliance rate.

What Are Monthly Replacement Contacts?

Most often, patients find monthly replacement contacts to be the most cost effective, comfortable option. Ocular health remains very high since patients find it easier to replace them on the first of each month. These lenses also do not require enzyme tablets, however like the two week lenses they must be cleaned and disinfected daily unless they are extended wear.

What Are Quarterly Replacement Contacts?

This category is usually reserved for patients with very high prescriptions or patients requiring custom contact lenses used in the treatment of non-refractive conditions such as keratoconus.

What Are Silicon Hydrogel Lenses?

The silicone hydrogel category represents the latest in soft contact lenses. Scientists found that by adding a small amount of silicone to the contact lens material they could greatly increase the oxygen transmissibility of the contact lenses. The problem; however, was that silicone is very hydrophobic, and the eye is a hydrophilic environment. Therefore, these lenses were quite uncomfortable. Eventually modern science prevailed, and a way was found to continue using the silicone, yet still make the lenses wettable and comfortable for the patient.

Now, the vast majority of extended wear contact lenses prescribed use the silicone hydrogel materials since it allows up to six times more air to reach the oxygen than the old materials.

What Can You Tell Me About Bifocal Contact Lenses?

Are you one of the millions of baby boomers who thought they had to give up contact lenses because they needed reading glasses?

Have you grown tired of taking your reading glasses on and off throughout the day?

Do you live an active lifestyle and find glasses inconvenient?

Bifocal contact lenses may be the answer for you. Why do I need bifocals is a common question. As children, we have a tremendous capacity to focus on objects that are close to us. As we get older our ability to focus on near objects slowly decreases to the point where around forty years of age we begin to notice that it takes a significant effort to read. We find that we need more light than we used to, the print quality has to be good and the font can't be too small, and we may notice that it's harder to read in the afternoon. Sometimes we can read at near, but when we look up, the distance is blurry. From the age of forty to approximately the mid sixties we notice the decline of our near vision. These are all signs of presbyopia (prez-be-'o-pe-a).

The good news is we have better options available than ever before. Bifocal contact lenses really do work. Progressive addition bifocal glasses also are better then they have ever been.

Bifocal contact lenses offer great lifestyle options. Bifocal contact lenses typically satisfy 60% to 80% of a patient's near point needs. Bifocal contact lenses improve a patient's lifestyle options by making it possible to do things like sign checks and read menus without reaching for their reading glasses. Without bifocal contacts, when someone hands you something to read, the first thing you do is look for your reading glasses or hold the reading material as far away from yourself as possible. If you are wearing your bifocal contact lenses you can probably read most material without reading glasses. You may need reading glasses for something small, such as taking a sliver out of a finger or reading the back of a medicine bottle. Fortunately, we don't do those things that often.

There are many types of bifocal contact lenses. Modern bifocal contact lenses are available in gas permeable and soft lens materials. We now have much more flexibility in our contact lens wearing schedules as well with daily disposable, two week, monthly, and quarterly replacement options. In the past, a patient with astigmatism would have to use reading glasses over their contacts or have to choose gas permeable bifocal contact lenses; however, now we even have soft bifocal toric contact lens that provide good, functional vision. Bifocal contact lenses have come a long way in recent years. Don't be afraid to give them a try.

What Is Monovision?

At some point, during our over forty years, we start to need some help to see near objects clearly. Many people hate the idea of wearing glasses and want another option. Monovision is a way to allow you to see at both distance and near.

One contact lens is used to make the distance clear in the dominant eye. In the other eye the power of the contact lens is altered, which will make the distance a little blurry and the near vision clearer. Thus one eye will allow you to see in the distance and the other eye will be used for near.

What Are The Pros And Cons To Monovision Contact Lenses?

The advantage to monovision is that we use regular contact lenses, thus it is a simple and inexpensive way to allow a person wearing contact lenses to see at distance and near without reading glasses.

The biggest disadvantage to monovision contact lenses is because you have one eye working at near and one at far, you will not have any depth perception, thus you may find it harder to judge distances to objects such as oncoming cars. A second disadvantage is that our visual system works best when both eyes are working together, so almost without exception we will experience our best vision when both of our eyes are working together. Therefore, patients wearing monovision contact lenses will not experience quite as good visual acuity at distance or near as they would have with both eyes corrected for distance, then wear reading glasses over their contact lenses.

Some patients simply cannot train their brain to adapt to monovision. The brain has to learn to ignore the blurry image from the eye that is not being used at the moment. For instance, if you are driving and your right eye is your distance eye, your left eye will be blurry. Some patients will experience a significant amount of eye strain as a result of this. Over a period of a few weeks their brain may be able to adapt by ignoring the blurry image.

Monovision is a good option for many patients. I find about 40% to 60% of patients are able to adapt to it. That said, bifocal contact lenses are usually my first choice in making my presbyopic patients glasses-free.

I Like My Monovision Contacts But How Can I Get Better Vision While Driving?

Many patients do well while wearing monovision contact lenses but don't feel safe wearing them while driving because their visual acuity isn't as sharp as they would like, or more often, they miss the lack of depth perception. Fortunately, there is a good solution to this dilemma. Many of us wear sunglasses while driving; therefore, problems with monovision can easily be fixed by wearing driving glasses over contact lenses. The glasses can be clear for night driving or made as sunglasses for daytime driving.

Monovision driving glasses essentially re-correct the near eye for distance, thus making both eyes now see well at distance, restoring your binocular vision.

My Eyes Don't Look The Same Can Contact Lenses Help?

Yes, those are called prosthetic contact lenses which use technology developed for the special effects film industry to make both eyes look the same. Prosthetic contact lenses can help people with severe corneal scarring, irregular pupils, and different colored eyes to achieve a more symmetric appearance.

Do UV Blocking Contact Lenses Really Work?

Johnson & Johnson, the parent company of Vistakon which makes the Acuvue line of contact lenses, conducted a study using rabbits and concluded that Ultraviolet (UV) absorbing contact lenses significantly reduced the UV-induced changes in the cornea, aqueous humor (fluid in the eye) and the lens. The study authors concluded that UV absorbent contact lenses were capable of protecting the cornea and crystalline lens of rabbit eyes from UV-induced changes.

So the question is, how does this affect humans? There are a number of contact lenses on the market today that block most of the UV rays. While we can't guarantee that the results of the study would apply to humans, we can generally infer that wearing this type of contact lens is beneficial for patients that spend a lot of time outdoors and do not wear sunglasses.

UV absorbent lenses do not protect our conjunctiva. The conjunctiva is the clear membrane that covers the blood vessels over the white part of the eye. This is an important reason as to why UV absorbent contact lenses are not a replacement for quality sunglasses. Excessive exposure to UV light on the conjunctiva is a leading cause for pterygia and pinguecula.

While not a replacement for good sunglasses, using UV absorbent contact lenses, especially in children, is a good practice.

Wearing Your Contacts Safely

What Is The Best Way To Clean My Contact Lens Case?

To prevent the contamination of your contact lens case, contact lens solution manufacturers recommend that you thoroughly rinse the entire empty contact lens case, including the lid or caps, with contact lens solution. Next, air dry your case by placing it upside-down on the counter in a way that allows air to circulate freely under it. A recent study determined that when these guidelines were followed, 82% of contact lens cases were contaminated with bacteria after one month. The same study also determined that if the cases were wiped down with a tissue after rinsing, the contamination rate was reduced to 72%.[15]

These rates appear to be unacceptably high as evidenced by another recent study indicating that wiping the contact lens case out with a tissue was three to four times more effective.[16] Surely there is a better way to disinfect our contact lens cases. Another frequent recommendation is to rinse the case with hot tap water, wipe it out, then allow the case to *thoroughly* air dry upside-down in a manner that would allow air to circulate around the case. It is difficult to thoroughly rinse a contact lens case with a fine stream of contact lens solution. When using contact lens solution to rinse the case, patients may not rinse the cases well in an effort to conserve solution.

My recommendation is to rinse the case with a strong stream of hot tap water, wipe the case out with a clean tissue, then allow the case to completely air dry in an upside-down position.

How Often Should I Replace My Contact Lens Case?

When was the last time you replaced your contact lens case? Next to dirty hands, contact lens cases are probably the most common source of bacteria that will contaminate your contact lenses. The best time to replace your contact lens case is when you get a new bottle of contact lens solution or every other month, whichever comes first. Better yet, make the move to daily disposable contact lenses and skip the contact lens case and solutions altogether.

What Is The Best Way To Clean My Contact Lenses?

A study out of Australia has confirmed what eye doctors have long suspected. Rubbing your contact lenses and briefly rinsing them prior, to overnight storage and disinfection is more effective at removing bacteria from the lens surface than merely placing the contacts in the case (no rub technique).[17] Numerous multipurpose no rub contact lens solutions have been approved by the FDA and shown to be an effective method of disinfecting contact lenses; however, this study shows that applying a few drops of the multipurpose solution, rubbing, then rinsing the lenses, is much more effective at removing bacteria from the lens surface.

This study was done "in-vitro," meaning that it was a lab study where patients did not actually wear these lenses, but the lenses were seeded with bacteria, then after the lenses were cleaned and disinfected, the lenses were tested to see how much bacteria was removed.

So the moral of the story is, after removing your soft contact lenses, add a few drops of the multipurpose contact lens solution, rub both sides of the lens, then rinse the lens and place it in the case to disinfect overnight.

I Wear My Contact Lenses Longer Than My Doctor Recommends, Is That Bad?

With the advent of disposable contact lenses, cases of Contact Lens Acute Red Eye (C.L.A.R.E) have been greatly reduced. The new generation of contact lens materials, known as the silicone hydrogels, have allowed extended wear contact lenses to make a resurgence. That said, wearing your contact lenses longer than your eye doctor and the FDA recommends puts you at a much greater risk for suffering contact lens related complications.

Can I Swim In My Contact Lenses?

It's a real killjoy to be invited to the beach or a swim party and not be able to see your friends because you have to squint to see anything beyond arm's length. It's true, you should not wear your regular contact lenses while swimming; however, daily disposable contact lenses are an excellent option to wear during water sports. Designed to be discarded at the end of each day, one day disposable contact lenses require no cleaning or disinfection, the next day you simply pop in another clean, brand new pair.

The risk with wearing your contact lenses to the beach or pool is that swimming pool water turns a contact lens into a bacteria magnet which you will then insert into your eye day after day, holding that bacteria-laden lens against your cornea until you retire those lenses for another pair. Soft contact lenses are essentially sponges, making an ideal medium for bacteria waiting for the right moment to attack your cornea.

How Can I Prevent Contact Lens Related Eye Infections?

The first thing, as stated above, is to not "stretch" your lenses, but replace them at the interval recommended by your eye doctor. Backup glasses are the next most important item. Having a pair of ten-year-old glasses that look like something Peggy Hill (from the TV series King of the Hill) would wear won't cut it. Your backup glasses should be glasses that you can wear comfortably, see well enough to pass a driver's test (20/30), and you don't mind being seen wearing them in public.

The incidence of vision loss as a result of contact lens wear has been greatly reduced. The chances of a patient losing vision as a result of extended wear contact lenses is actually less than the rate of permanent vision loss from LASIK.

Why Should Contact Lens Wearers Have Backup Glasses?

Almost all contact lens wearers feel like "I wear contacts because I don't like glasses." Then why is it important for everyone to have backup glasses? The simple answer is that your eyes need a break. The incidence of eye infections in contact lens wearers is much lower for patients who have an adequate backup pair of glasses.

A contact lens wearers that lack a pair of backup glasses will have to wear their contacts when their eyes are red and irritated, thus never giving their eyes a chance to fully recover. Most contact lens-related eye irritations will resolve in less than a day if the contacts are not worn. Wearing your backup glasses at the first sign of a mild eye irritation can prevent a mild irritation from becoming a full blown ulcer. If your eye is not back to 100% within one day or is light-sensitive at any time, you should call your eye doctor.

What Are Backup Eye Glasses?

What qualifies a pair of eyeglasses as backup glasses? Here is what I think is important.:

- The frame and lens styles are not so out of date that you don't mind being seen wearing them in public.

- You can see well enough with them to pass your driver's test (20/30 or better), and last but not least, the most important one . . .

- You can find them.

How Do I Make Homemade Saline For My Contact Lenses?

Please don't do this. Making your own contact lens solution has not been recommended since the early eighties. Modern contact lens solutions are safe and effective. Thankfully, reports of true contact lens solution related allergies are now extremely rare. There is no reason any longer to make your own saline solution. The incidence of severe corneal ulcers is the highest among patients using homemade saline.

Top 10 DO's For Successful Contact Lens Wear

Here are the top 10 recommendations for successful contact lens wear from the FDA with some embellishments on my part.

1. Always wash your hands before handling your contact lenses.

2. Remove your contact lenses immediately if your eyes are red or irritated. Conversely, do not insert your contact lenses if your eyes are red, irritated, or light sensitive.

3. Always follow the instructions of your eye doctor. She has selected your contact lens solutions and contact lenses to improve your chances of wearing contact lenses successfully.

4. Use contact lens solutions that are recommended by your eye doctor.

5. After removing your contact lenses, clean them by rubbing and rinsing them, even if you are using a "no rub" contact lens solution.

6. Clean and disinfect your contact lenses properly by following all of the directions on your contact lens products.

7. Clean and disinfect your contact lens case after every use.

8. Replace your contact lens case at least every three months

9. Have a pair of backup glasses

10. Have a pair of backup contact lenses.

Top 10 Contact Lens DON'Ts For Successful Contact Lens Wear

Again, these are from the FDA with some additional recommendations on my part.

1. Don't use expired contact lens products.

2. Don't save contact lens solution from the prior day and top it off.

3. Don't store your lenses in tap water or distilled water.

4. Don't put your contact lenses in your mouth to clean or temporarily store them. *Eeeeewwwww!*

5. When preparing to travel, don't transfer contact lens solution to a smaller "travel" bottle. Your eye doctor often has travel size bottles of contact lens solutions available.

6. Don't purchase store brand contact lens solutions. The contents/vendors of those solutions are not consistent over time or purchase location, ie. You don't know what you are getting. In addition, store bought brands are not the latest formulation. The store brand's cola doesn't taste like a Coke nor are the store brand contact lens solutions equivalent to the name brand solutions.

7. Don't s t r e c h your contact lens replacement schedule. One red eye will wipe-out many years of "savings," plus it hurts . . . a lot.

8. Don't wear a damaged contact lens as it will scratch the cornea, greatly increasing the chances of a bacterial corneal ulcer.

9. Don't wear someone else's contact lenses . . . Double *eeeeeeeewwwwww*!

10. Don't sleep in contact lenses intended for daily wear only. If you want to sleep in contact lenses, ask your eye doctor for different contacts. There are many options that will allow you to safely do this.

Orthokeratology, Corneal Molding, Ortho-K, and Vision Shaping Treatment

Orthokeratology, also commonly known as corneal refractive therapy, vision shaping treatment, corneal molding, and Ortho-K, is the gentle reshaping of the cornea to correct myopia (nearsightedness). Research is also being done on using corneal reshaping in the treatment of hyperopia, though like the use of LASIK for the treatment of hyperopia, the results are not as consistent or predictable.

I believe that some of the current research into slowing or stopping the progression of myopia with OrthoKeratology will change how we treat nearsightedness in children. This is an area of great potential.

What Is The History of Ortho-K? – How Was It Started?

Orthokeratology is known by numerous names, and the technique has changed greatly over the years. Various forms of Ortho-k have been practiced for about forty years. The technique first involved using progressively flatter lenses to flatten the cornea, causing the patient to become less nearsighted. This early method required months to show results, required numerous lens changes, and the patients had to wear their lenses during part of each day or on alternating days.

Corneal Molding has evolved into a method where over 80% of the patients achieve success with the first pair of lenses. Good results typically take less than a week. The process is accomplished while the patient sleeps, often using a computer designed reverse geometry contact lens. The lenses are inserted at bedtime and removed in the morning. The lenses, also known as vision retainers, safely and gently reshape the cornea, changing the eye's focus. Most patients will have good vision throughout the day. Some patients may only need to wear their lenses on alternate nights to maintain good vision.

How Does Modern OrthoKeratology Work?

Orthokeratology is accomplished by using a specially designed contact lens called a reverse geometry lens that gently flattens the cornea by pushing and pulling the central epithelial layers that reside directly over the pupil toward the periphery (shown in Figure 19 below). This movement of corneal cells causes the center of the cornea to be thinner, thus moving the focus of light closer to the retina. Orthokeratology refocuses the light on the retina in the same way as LASIK and PRK.

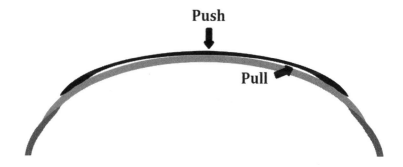

Figure 19   Cross Section OrthoK Lens on The Eye

Below are corneal topography images. The image on the left is a normal cornea before wearing Ortho-K lenses. The middle image is the same patient after wearing OrthoKeratology lenses. The red ring shows the epithelial cells that were in the center and have now been pulled to the periphery. The image to the right shows how the corneal topography looks after LASIK (different patient).

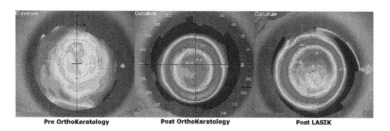

Pre OrthoKeratology   Post OrthoKeratology   Post LASIK

Figure 20   Corneal Topography Before & After OrthoK and with LASIK

What Kind Of Training Is Required Of Doctors Fitting Overnight Orthokeratology Lenses?

The traditional methods of fitting the reverse geometry lenses used in modern Ortho-K do not follow traditional contact lens fitting methods. Because of this difference, the FDA restricts the use of these lenses to only those doctors who have been specially trained in their use. This is an additional requirement that has never been used for contact lenses; however, it is much like the requirement for the additional training required of physicians who use the excimer laser for LASIK and PRK.

Are there Different Names for Orthokeratology?

Yes, there are a number of different names for orthokeratology, orthoK, corneal molding, corneal reshaping, and corneal refractive therapy are some of the most common names.

Is Overnight OrthoKeratology FDA Approved?

Yes, a handful of orthokeratology lenses have been approved for overnight orthokeratology by the FDA., most notably, lenses from Baush & Lomb that employ the Vision Shaping Treatment® such as the DreamLens® and the Paragon CRT Lens (Corneal Refractive Therapy) from Paragon Systems. The Wave Contact Lens System attained FDA approval in late 2011.

Is Orthokeratology Safe?

Yes, Orthokeratology has been shown to be a safe and effective means of reducing nearsightedness. It is just one of the many options, including LASIK, PRK, soft contact lenses, and glasses that are available to patients.[18]

What Are My Vision Correction Options?

Expect your eye doctor to consult with you regarding the wide range of options available to you. He or she will help you focus on which option or options best fulfill your visual needs.

Glasses

This is the most common, safest, and simplest option. All contact lens wearers should have a pair of glasses that they can fall back on when they cannot or should not be wearing their contact lenses.

Traditional Contact Lenses

Traditional contact lenses provide a number of options with variable replacement schedules from soft contact lenses that are discarded daily, every two weeks, or monthly. There are also contact lenses that can be safely worn overnight from six nights to as many as thirty consecutive nights. Studies have shown that contact lens wear, even considering a lifetime of wear, is safer than refractive surgery[19]. Both soft and gas permeable lenses can correct high amounts of nearsightedness, astigmatism, and farsightedness. Contact lenses can also correct presbyopia, allowing patients over forty to see at both near and far without bifocal glasses or reading glasses.

Refractive surgery

Refractive surgery is a popular option for reducing a patient's dependency on glasses; however, not everyone is a candidate for refractive surgery. The most popular refractive procedure is LASIK or Laser **AS**sisted **I**n situ **K**eratomileusis; however, PRK, or Photo Refractive Keratectomy, is still popular. Non-laser refractive surgeries such as Clear Lensectomy or Refractive Lensectomy and Implantable Contact Lenses are also available; however, they are not nearly as popular as LASIK and PRK. There are a number of reasons why a person may not be a candidate for LASIK or PRK. For more information on refractive surgery, see page 95.

Why Not Have LASIK Instead Of Orthokeratology?

The most common contraindications to refractive surgery are large pupil size, thin corneas, occupation, refractive error, surgical expectations and age. In addition, some patients simply are not comfortable with having surgery on their eyes or are hesitant to undertake something such as LASIK or PRK that is permanent.

Who Is A Good Orthokeratology Candidate?

- The moderately nearsighted

- Children

- Adults

- Children who have experienced a sharp increase in nearsightedness

- Patients afraid to have elective surgery on their eyes

- Athletes

- Patients denied refractive surgery due to occupation

- People with a fear of, or anxiety toward, eye surgery
- Patients who can't wear contact lenses due to dry eyes

What Are The Advantages To OrthoKeratology?

- Safer than refractive surgery
- Works while you sleep
- Much better solution for patients with dry eyes
- Studies show it prevents the progression of nearsightedness in children
- It's reversible
- Proven technique for over forty years

What Are The Disadvantages To OrthoKeratology?

- Risk of vision-threatening eye infection similar to that of traditional contact lens wearers, though many times less than the complication rate experienced by LASIK patients
- Possible halos at night
- Fluctuating vision

It is good to know that, because Ortho-K is reversible, symptoms that you may experience such as halos and fluctuating vision are reversible.

What Should I Expect At An Orthokeratology Consult?

Most orthokeratologists will offer a free Ortho-K consult for patients interested in Ortho-K. If the patient is an orthokeratology candidate and wishes to proceed, the next step is a comprehensive eye exam and an orthokeratology contact lens evaluation. The initial orthokeratology evaluation will involve corneal topography along with a consultation discussing how orthokeratology works and what to expect.

During the initial consultation, the doctor may begin to evaluate the fit of diagnostic lenses on your eyes, using the corneal topography data to determine which contact lens parameters will safely flatten your cornea, resulting in clearer vision. Alternatively, the initial lenses can be designed empirically from testing data collected at the consultation. Both methods work well, and your doctor will determine which method is best for you.

After your doctor receives your new contact lenses and the lens parameters are verified, your doctor's office will call you to schedule a time to dispense your contacts, teach you how to insert, remove and care for your new lenses.

How Are Ortho-K Lenses Worn?

Since 2002, when various Ortho-K lens manufacturers proved to the FDA's satisfaction that Ortho-K lenses could be safely worn at night, the typical wear schedule involves inserting your lenses right before bedtime, then removing them when you wake up.

What Is Corneal Topography And Why Is It Important?

Corneal topography gives your doctor detailed shape information of your cornea by showing all of the different corneal curves. Everyone's corneal topography map is different, much like our fingerprints. Corneal topography is essential in treating corneal conditions such as keratoconus and fitting patients with contact lenses to correct problems that resulted as a complication to refractive surgery or corneal transplants. Corneal topography is also essential to designing orthokeratology contact lenses that will mold your cornea. Corneal conditions such as keratoconus and pellucid marginal degeneration are diagnosed using a corneal topographer.

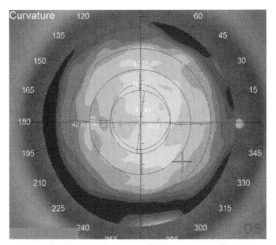

Normal Corneal Topography

Figure 21   Normal Corneal Topography

Facts About Contact Lenses

Who Invented Soft Contact Lenses?

The first soft contact lens material was developed by the Czech chemists Otto Wichterle and Drahoslav Lim in the late 1950s.

How Long Have Soft Contacts Been Around?

The first soft hydrogel contact lens to be approved by the FDA in the US was Bausch & Lomb's *Soflens* in 1971.

What Are The Benefits Of Contact Lenses For Children?

According to a three-year study of children ages eight to eleven years old, young contact lens wearers felt better about their physical appearance, athletic competence, and social acceptance. The study showed that, in short, contact lenses improved the self-image of children.[20,21] Most children become contact lens wearers in their early teen years, an uncertain time for children where they begin to spend a lot more time among their peers and are just beginning to emerge from the constant supervision of their parents.

In addition to helping children with social acceptance, contact lenses also help athletic performance. Contact lenses provide a more natural form of vision correction, improving a young athlete's peripheral vision. It is hard to play a sport with dirty lenses and glasses that steam up or slide down on your face. Generally, it is a very bad idea for children to play sports with their regular glasses. And some sports, such as racquet sports, should always be played with athletic eyewear. As children get older, athletic completion increases, optimal vision correction becomes an important part of maximizing a child's athletic performance.

How Do I Know When My Child Is Ready For Contact Lenses?

I find that, unless the contact lenses are medically necessary, responsibility is the most important requirement before introducing a child to contact lenses. The motivation to wear contact lenses, however, is also important. If children have to be regularly reminded to take care of basic hygiene needs, such as taking a shower and brushing their teeth then they probably aren't ready to handle the responsibilities of contact lenses on their own.

Can Contact Lenses Be Used to Deliver Medication?

Currently, there are no FDA approved contact lenses to do so; however, it is expected that this option will be available in the United States soon. There have been reports of contact lenses being used to administer stem cell therapy outside of the US.

Should I Buy My Contact Lenses From My Eye Doctor?

We all think it is important not to spend our money foolishly and, therefore, we want to get the most bang for our buck. It is not uncommon for us to be asked, "Why should I buy contact lenses from my eye doctor?" In David Letterman style, here are the top 10 reasons why you might want to buy your contacts from your eye doctor:

1. You are guaranteed to get the correct lenses in the correct parameters.

2. You are guaranteed to get unexpired lenses.

3. If your lenses are not performing properly, you don't have to worry about exchanging your old lenses. Your local eye doctor wants you to be a happy, successful contact lens wearer. If your contact lenses aren't working out for you, your eye doctor is going to want to do what it takes to make you successful.

4. Should your prescription change, you can usually exchange unopened, unexpired, or unmarked boxes in new condition.

5. If you have a defective contact lens or lose a lens, your doctor will likely replace it for you for free.

6. Contact lens companies are rebate happy. Rebates typically run between $30 to $100 for a one year supply of contacts. Your eye doctor will have the latest manufacturer's rebates available to save you money.

7. Patient satisfaction is highest when patients can purchase their contact lenses from the doctor who prescribed them. If there is a problem, there is no middle man to point a finger at, thus your doctor will offer competitive pricing.

8. Whether the lenses are delivered to your home or work or you stop by your doctor's office, the shipping is typically free.

9. You will be getting the lenses from an authorized distributor of the brand you wear.

10. You will have the satisfaction of supporting a local business that cares about you and your eyes. Things happen; if something doesn't go according to plan, it's nice to be able to talk to someone in person rather than over email or a person manning a phone bank on the other side of the country or, worse yet, in another country.

Dr. Richard A Driscoll

CHAPTER EIGHT

Refractive Surgery

Here is another top fiver in the most frequently asked questions department. In the office, patients most often want to know if they are a candidate. However, when I meet people outside of the office and they know that I'm an eye doctor, they want to know what I think about LASIK, PRK, or clear lens extraction etc. In a nutshell, refractive surgery is a perfect example of how patients should do their research and be well informed before getting a consult. Refractive surgery is a big step. You only have two eyes and, to paraphrase Gene Kranz, NASA Flight Director of Apollo 13, *"Replacement is not an option."*

The Facts On Laser Vision Correction

What Is The History Of The Excimer Laser?

The excimer laser was invented in Russia in 1970. Researchers at IBM noted that the excimer laser could make clean ablations in man-made materials without disrupting the surrounding tissue and thought that maybe it could do the same for living tissue. The day after Thanksgiving 1981 one of the researchers, Rangaswamy Srinivasan, brought some leftover Thanksgiving turkey and found that he was able to burn clean patterns in the meat, bone, and cartilage without disrupting the adjacent tissue. Two years later in the summer of 1983, Dr. Stephen Trokel, an ophthalmologist with

Columbia Presbyterian Medical Center in New York City, worked with the researchers at IBM to see if the excimer laser might be used for eye surgery. Their work resulted in a published paper, and in 1995 the excimer laser achieved FDA approval for ophthalmic surgery.

The excimer laser has been instrumental in advancing the high technology industry where it is used to engrave silicon chips used in electronics.

Is Laser Vision Correction Safe?

The FDA has determined that Laser Vision Correction is a safe and effective means of treating myopia, hyperopia, or astigmatism.

Which Is Safer LASIK Or Contact Lenses?

It's all over the radio these days. A LASIK surgeon touts "Some experts believe LASIK is safer than contact lenses." In reality, this is a difficult statement to back up properly, given that we are comparing apples to oranges. Why is this comparison difficult? Comparing LASIK to another refractive surgery procedure, such as PRK, is rather straightforward because the complications are similar for both procedures and the opportunity for complications is essentially nil after the patient is stable, typically six months to a year after surgery. A contact lens wearer, on the other hand, has a much lower complication rate spread over a greater amount of time. When compared to LASIK or PRK, contact lens complications are less severe and less frequent; however, a contact lens wearer's potential for complications will last as long as the patient is wearing their lenses, often for decades.

Both LASIK and contact lenses are safe options. The key to successful vision correction is finding an eye doctor who has experience with all forms of vision correction. A qualified eye care consultant should be able to offer spectacle, contact lens, orthokeratology and refractive surgery options to you. Your consultant should inform you of the pros and cons of all the options available. With this information you can then intelligently weigh the risks and benefits of all alternatives before proceeding.

As a practical matter, the incidence of vision-threatening problems in compliant as well as non-compliant contact lens wearers is small. When patients have a problem, it typically manifests itself as a red eye, usually resulting from poor care or not replacing their contact lenses as often as recommended. It is exceedingly rare for a contact lens-related red eye to cause a patient to require surgery to resolve the problem.

This prompts me to ask "what does the research say?" In my mind that's what matters. Let the studies show us which is safer. The most important contact lens and LASIK complications are those that have resulted in a loss of vision; therefore, that is the best criteria to compare LASIK versus extended wear contact lenses. The 2005 study referenced earlier by Schein included almost 5,000 patients followed over a one year period showed that thirty day Ciba Night & Day contact lens wearers experienced an overall rate of presumed infiltrative keratitis (a type of corneal ulcer) of 0.18%. Of those experiencing keratitis, 0.036% resulted in a loss of vision and 0.144% experienced keratitis without vision loss.[19]

Numerous studies published in 2005 and 2006 indicated a complication rate for LASIK, resulting in a loss of best corrected vision ranging from 0.6% to 7.0%.

Given the facts outlined above, I feel it is doing patients a disservice to state or imply that refractive surgery is as safe or safer than silicone hydrogel contact lenses. Both LASIK/PRK and silicone hydrogel contact lenses have come a long way in reducing both the rate and severity of complications and, in looking at the numbers, both are safe.

LASIK and PRK are good options for patients and as such they remain one of the treatment options, along with the others listed above, that I recommend for my patients. However, the research does not support the statement that refractive surgery is as safe or safer than contact lens wear nor should it be promoted as such.

What Are The Long-Term Effects Of LASIK?

Excimer laser procedures have been prevalent in many countries around the world since the late 1980's. Many clinical studies have investigated the long-term effects (fifteen years) of the Excimer laser on the cornea. All of these studies, without exception, have failed to demonstrate any long-term negative effects on the integrity of the eye. Patients who require an enhancement procedure or develop a complication will typically do so within the first few months following the procedure, not years later.

It is essential that you understand as much as possible about the risks associated with the Excimer laser procedure. The risk of having a serious vision-threatening complication is less than 1% according to the Eye Surgery Education Council. The Excimer laser procedure, however, like all surgical procedures, has limitations and risks. Your doctor will go over all of these risks in great detail with you and will encourage you to ask questions.

Will I Have Perfect Vision After The Procedure?

Experience has shown us that Laser Vision Correction has been overwhelmingly successful in significantly reducing nearsightedness (myopia), farsightedness (hyperopia), and astigmatism. While vision improves significantly following the procedure, the degree of improvement may vary between patients. Overall, studies have shown that almost 100% of nearsighted patients achieve 20/40 vision or better, which means they can drive legally, enjoy sports, and join the police or fire departments, all without their glasses. The visual outcome largely depends on their degree of pre-surgical nearsightedness. Generally, of the patients under -7.00, 98% were 20/20 at the one year mark and 100% were 20/40 or better. For the highly nearsighted, the results are also good, with 86% achieving 20/20. The more nearsighted you are, the greater the chance that you will experience complications and regression (some of your nearsightedness returning).

Will I Still Need My Glasses?

For distance, you probably won't need glasses. If you are over forty, I would count on needing them to read.

Will LASIK Fix My Need for Reading Glasses?

Laser vision surgery will not affect the progression of presbyopia. You will still need reading glasses after LASIK or any refractive surgery. If you are in your forties or older you will most likely require reading glasses after laser vision correction surgery. The need for reading glasses would be present regardless of whether you have laser vision correction surgery or not; however, when we are nearsighted, we get around the need for reading glasses or extend the time before reading glasses are necessary by removing our glasses to read.

What Is Monovision LASIK?

Monovision LASIK is where one eye, usually your non dominant eye, is under corrected so patients over forty can read without glasses. Monovision LASIK works better for those who are just starting to need reading glasses. The older we get, the more help we need to make our near vision clear; therefore, the greater amount of under correction that is needed.

The more under correction, the greater the distance blur, thus the bigger difference there is in vision between the eyes. All of the advantages and disadvantages for monovision with LASIK also apply to contact lenses (please see the Monovision section for a detailed discussion). In short, a small degree of under correction, say 0.75D, may be tolerable. The biggest disadvantage to monovision LASIK is that it is permanent and the near vision needs of 45 year olds are much different than that of a 55-year-old. Monovision in contact lenses is not permanent and, when you need good binocular vision, driving at night on a rainy road, for instance, (I know you'll never be in that situation; you never drive at night ;-)) you can take your lenses out and put in the backup glasses we talked about earlier. With monovision LASIK corrections above the -0.75D we talked about earlier, the difference between the two eyes does not lend itself well to wearing glasses, with patients experiencing significant eyestrain and often headaches.

Before you undergo monovision LASIK, I would highly recommend you try monovision contact lenses for at least a month simulating the correction the surgeon intends for you.

Does The Procedure Hurt?

No, the procedure is painless. Most LASIK patients experience only some irritation (usually reported as a burning sensation), light sensitivity, and watering of their eyes for a day or two. For PRK patients I recommend that you closely stick to the drop regiment prescribed by your doctor. The recovery for a PRK patient is longer than that for a LASIK patient (often three to four days) and PRK patients usually experience more discomfort. Sticking to the drop regimen even if your eyes feel great will maximize your comfort during this period.

Can Anyone Have LASIK? Am I A Candidate?

LASIK and PRK will not work for everyone; however, most nearsighted patients are candidates, as well as many patients with astigmatism and farsightedness. The best way to determine if you are a candidate for refractive surgery is to schedule a consult with your doctor so she can cover all of the options with you.

Does Insurance Cover The Costs Of Laser Vision Correction?

Typically, no. Very few insurance companies will cover refractive surgery. Insurance companies usually look at refractive surgery as an elective procedure. However, many employers have "flex accounts" or cafeteria plans for unreimbursed medical expenses. A flex account allows you to use before tax dollars to pay for medical expenses that were not covered by your insurance plan. Flex plans cover laser vision correction as a reimbursable expense.

Are Payment Plans Available For LASIK Surgery?

Most offices offer numerous forms of payment, such as credit cards, flexible spending accounts, health savings accounts, and financing.

What Do The Fees For Refractive Surgery Include?

Typically your refractive surgery fees will include a consultation with the surgeon, your preoperative and postoperative care. Some doctors will include enhancements as well for a specified period of time, usually six to twelve months.

Will My Nearsightedness Return After Surgery?

It is highly unlikely that you will return to your previous correction; however, regression after laser vision correction is not uncommon, though it is easily corrected with an enhancement, contact lenses, or glasses. Often the degree of regression is minimal, and patients who wish to return their vision back to the prior level but do not want to undergo retreatment will opt to occasionally wear glasses, especially for driving.

Can I Wear My Contact Lenses Before The Procedure?

The use of contact lenses directly affects the shape and hydration of the cornea. Therefore, it is necessary to remove contact lenses prior to both the pre-operative eye exam and prior to your surgery.

Soft contact lens wearers should remove their contact lenses one to two weeks prior to both pre-operative exam and surgery.

Rigid contact lenses (gas permeable and standard hard lenses) should be removed approximately six weeks prior to both the pre-operative examination and surgery. Many patients are unwilling to wear glasses for this long; therefore, they are often refit with soft contact lenses to help with the transition. It is important not to be in a hurry to have surgery following cessation of rigid contact lens wear. Having laser vision correction surgery before the cornea is stable will increase the likelihood of an enhancement being necessary.

How do I Find A Good Place To Have My Laser Vision Correction Surgery?

This is probably the most important step in your search for vision correction. If you have an eye doctor who you trust and stays on top of the latest developments in eye care, then that is without question your best source of information. Recommendations from friends, family, and co-workers would be a distant second choice.

So why does it seem that I am not holding friends, family, and co-workers as a better resource for laser vision correction recommendations when referrals from this same group drives the growth of most, if not all, successful practices? Recommendations from people you know can be a great resource; however what is of more value is getting the recommendation from a doctor who has seen the surgical results from many different surgeons. If you already have an eye doctor you know and trust, especially if it's an optometrist who is not directly involved in the surgery then he or she can advise you on the pros and cons of all of your vision correction options rather than merely telling you whether you are a candidate for laser vision correction. Surgical correction may or may not be an option for you. Your family eye doctor wants what is best for you. He or she should present you with all of your options in an unbiased manner.

"Yes, but my optometrist will lose me as a patient if I elect to have refractive surgery; therefore, he will probably advise me against it." Your family eye doctor will still be seeing you and your family for regular eye care. You may not need glasses or contact lenses; however, you still should have yearly eye exams. A yearly eye exam evaluates not only your vision, but more importantly the health of your eye. Nearsighted patients have a higher incidence of retinal detachments. Even if a patient has had refractive surgery, the risk for retinal detachment has not changed. The only way to adequately evaluate this risk is with a yearly dilated eye exam.

Should I Go Directly To The Surgeon For The LASIK?

That is one option. However, if you go to a Chevy dealer, the only choice is a Chevy. If you go to a doctor who works with multiple surgeons, he or she can recommend which surgical team she feels would be best for you.

Should I Consult My Optometrist About My Refractive Surgery Options?

A patient who elects to go directly to the refractive surgeon will most likely receive the pre and post-op care from a technician. One of the most important pieces of data calculated during the pre-op evaluation is your prescription. Your prescription is the cornerstone to achieving a good result. Yes, technicians can be taught to determine your prescription; however, this key piece of data is probably best left to someone with considerable experience in managing a patient's refractive needs.

An optometrist is independent of the laser center. Your eye doctor is your advocate, wanting the best possible surgical outcome for you. His goal is to collect the most accurate refractive data for programming the laser, then work with a laser center that will follow through on your eye doctor's mission of providing you the best possible chance of a successful outcome.

Refractive Surgery Options

What Are My Surgical Options For Vision Correction?

The most common refractive surgery options are LASIK, PRK, LASEK, IntraLase, Implantable Contact Lenses, Refractive Lensectomy, and Intacs

What Is LASIK?

Laser **AS**sisted **I**n-situ **K**eratomileusis, or LASIK, is the most common refractive surgery today and involves using a device called a microkeratome to make a thin flap of the cornea (through the epithelium and the upper layers of the stroma) that remains attached in one quadrant. The flap is then pulled back, and a computer-controlled excimer laser is then used to reshape the cornea. Once the laser computer program is complete, the corneal surgeon unfolds the flap, tapes the eye closed, and repeats the process on the other eye.

What Is The Real Scoop On LASIK?

Pros

- Relatively quick recovery time of one to two days

- Minimal discomfort

- Proven, reliable technology. Lasers used in LASIK gained FDA approval in 1998

Cons

- Not recommended for large pupil sizes

- Not for thin corneas

What Is PRK?

Photo Refractive Keratectomy, or PRK, is still quite popular. Essentially, PRK is similar to LASIK except no flap is made. Instead, the epithelial cells are either scraped away or vaporized during the laser treatment. After the laser program is complete, a bandage contact lens is then applied to the eye. The contact lens serves to aid healing and reduce discomfort. The contact lens will remain in the eye until the corneal epithelium regrows over the cornea, usually three or four days. It is not uncommon for the complete visual recovery to take one to two weeks.

What's The 411 On PRK?

Pros

- Better than LASIK for thinner corneas

- Generally, safer option since no flap is made

- Proven, reliable technology, gained FDA approval in 1995

Cons

- Moderate discomfort lessening over three to seven days

- Visual recovery may take up to two to three weeks

- Not recommended for large pupils

What Is IntraLase?

Also known as IntraLASIK or ILASIK; IntraLase is essentially the same as LASIK except for an important distinction in how the flap is created. While LASIK uses a steel blade to make a thick flap of corneal tissue, IntraLASIK uses a femtosecond laser to make a thin flap. The specifications of this flap are computer-controlled, allowing for much greater control over the depth, diameter, and shape. It remains to be seen whether LASIK or IntraLASIK give better visual outcomes.

What are The Pros and Cons of IntraLASIK?

Pros

- Can treat thinner corneas than LASIK because the flap parameters can be tightly controlled

- Fewer complications related to flap creation

- Proven, reliable technology, gained FDA approval in 2001

Cons

- Longer recovery than LASIK, but less than PRK

- More post-surgical discomfort than LASIK

- Slightly more expensive than LASIK or PRK

What Is LASEK?

Laser Epithelial Keratomileusis is a combination of both LASIK and PRK. Instead of using a flat oscillating blade to make a corneal flap, a circular blade called a trephine (it looks like a short can attached to a handle with the top and bottom cut out) is used to cut through the corneal epithelium. While the trephine is in place a 20% alcohol solution is placed inside the well of the trephine for thirty seconds. The purpose of the alcohol solution is to cause the corneal epithelium to separate from the corneal stroma. Once the epithelium has separated, it is then folded back on the hinged side (side that was not cut, just like in LASIK) and the computer-controlled excimer laser vaporizes the exposed corneal tissue. Once the computer controlled-program is complete, the epithelium is then unfolded and repositioned over the treatment zone. A bandage contact lens is then applied and left in place for a few days.

What are The Pros and Cons of LASEK?

Pros

- Better for thinner corneas
- Preferred over LASIK for scars on the front of the cornea
- Generally, safer than LASIK since neither a laser nor blade are used to make a flap
- Proven, reliable technology
- Preserves corneal nerves, thus reducing laser surgery-related dry eye symptoms

Cons

- Moderate discomfort lessening over two to four days
- Visual recovery may take up to ten to fourteen days
- The use of alcohol to separate and lift the epithelium is toxic to the epithelium, prolonging recovery and increasing post surgical discomfort

What Is Epi-LASIK?

Epi-LASIK is a cross between LASIK and LASEK. Both Epi-LASIK and LASEK make a flap containing only the epithelium. LASEK uses a trephine blade (it looks like a tube that is sharp on one end which allows the surgeon to make a circular incision) and alcohol to separate and lift the epithelium; however, in Epi-LASIK an epi-keratome is used to make a flap containing only the corneal epithelium. Once the epithelial flap is made and folded back, the exposed corneal stroma is then treated with the excimer laser as in LASIK. The flap is then repositioned and a bandage contact lens is applied.

What are The Pros and Cons of Epi-LASEK?

Pros

- Better option for thinner corneas
- Faster recovery time than with LASEK since it does not use alcohol, thus preserving the viability of the epithelium
- Preferred over LASIK for scars on the front of the cornea
- Longstanding technique, developed in 2003
- Preserves corneal nerves, thus reducing laser related dry eye symptoms

Cons

- Moderate discomfort lessening over two to four days
- Visual recovery may take up to ten to fourteen days

What Are Implantable Contact Lens?

The implantable contact lens (ICL), or phakic IOLs, is just like it says, a lens that is inserted into the eye in front of the natural ocular lens. There are currently two different ICLs. The Visian ICL is placed behind the iris, but in front of the ocular lens. The Verisyse ICL is attached to the front of the iris. The implantable contact lenses are more often used for patients who have very high refractive errors, making them poor candidates for the laser vision correction procedures. Because implantable contact lenses require intra-ocular surgery that carries with it a higher complication, rate they are best used in patients who are not a candidate for one of the other procedures.

What are The Pros and Cons of Implantable Contact Lenses?

Pros

- Less likely to cause night vision problems caused by large pupil size

- Independent of corneal thickness

- Good for cases of extreme myopia (we are talking myopia in the double digits here)

- Preserves corneal nerves, thus an alternative for patients with severe dry eyes

- Procedure is reversible

- Rapid recovery; vision improves immediately

Cons

- Increased risk of cataracts

- Increased risk of retinal detachment

- Increased risk of glaucoma

- Reversal of procedure requires surgery

What Is A Refractive Lensectomy?

Also known by a number of other names such as refractive lens exchange, clear lens exchange, and clear lens extraction, this refractive surgery option involves removing the eye's natural lens and replacing it with an intra ocular lens, refocusing the light on the macula for clearer vision. Better candidates for refractive lensectomy are typically over fifty, may have early cataracts or are farsighted.

What are The Pros and Cons of Refractive Lensectomy?

Pros

- Less likely to cause night vision problems caused by large pupil size

- Works well for thin corneas

- Good for cases of extreme myopia (we are talking double digits here)

- Preserves corneal nerves, thus an alternative for patients with severe dry eyes

Cons

- Increased risk of retinal detachment

- Increased risk of glaucoma

- Not reversible

- Not recommended for patients under 45

- Candidate selection is important

What Can You Tell Me About Intacs?

Intacs were originally approved for correcting myopia of -1.00 to -3.00 diopters; however, it was soon replaced by better procedures such as LASIK and PRK. Intacs involves taking two small pieces of curved plastic (uses the same material as hard contact lenses) that are shaped like parentheses and inserting them within the cornea (no small feat since the cornea is only ½ mm thick) at the edge of the pupil with one being on the right and one on the left, just like opposing parentheses. Intacs is rarely used now for refractive surgery since other better procedures exist today.

What are The Pros and Cons of Intacs?

Pros

- Less likely to cause night vision problems caused by large pupil size

- Independent of corneal thickness

- Procedure is reversible

Cons

- Requires higher degree of surgical skill

- Limited treatment range

- More expensive than other procedures

- Reversal of procedure requires surgery

What Are My Non-Surgical Options For Vision Correction?

- Eyeglasses, the old reliable, newer lens materials are thinner, lighter and much more scratch resistant than ever before. For more information, see page 173.

- Orthokeratology, an FDA approved method discussed in greater detail on page 83, Ortho-K involves wearing contact lenses that remold your cornea while you sleep. Upon waking, they are removed and the patient sees clearly. Ortho-K is reversible.

- Contact lenses, extended wear contact lenses vary from those that you discard daily to those that can be worn continuously for up to thirty days. Additional information on contact lenses can be found on page 68.

What Is Radial Keratotomy?

Radial Keratotomy is a surgical procedure developed in the 1970's by Russian ophthalmologist, Dr. Svyatoslav Fyodorov. Also known by its acronym RK, the procedure involves using a diamond scalpel to make incisions that start from just inside the white part of the eye toward the center. The incisions are usually about 4 mm long, extend through 90% of the corneal thickness, and stop before reaching the center of the cornea. The central 4 mm of the cornea are left untouched. Most patients receive either four or eight incisions, as in the diagram below.

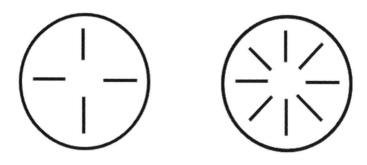

Figure 22   Radial Keratotomy, 4 incision and 8 incision

Radial Keratotomy is used to reduce a patient's nearsightedness. RK was introduced into the United States in 1978 and was a popular ophthalmic surgical procedure throughout the 1980's. With the advent of the excimer laser, RK quickly fell out of favor in the mid to early 1990's and was replaced by PRK, photo refractive keratectomy.

Why Is Radial Keratotomy No Longer Popular?

There are a number of reasons why RK fell out of favor. PRK, with the excimer laser, being a much safer and more reliable procedure was the primary reason. The recovery time for radial keratotomy was often as long as a week where the patient usually experienced significant pain and light sensitivity. The surgical results from RK were often unpredictable, and the retreatment or enhancement rate was high. Because the incisions weakened the patient's cornea, patients often experienced fluctuating vision.

Changes in altitude would also cause significant changes in a person's vision. Altitude-induced vision changes were experienced by Dr. Beck Weathers in 1996 when he attempted to climb Mount Everest. Glare was also a significant problem with RK. In my experience, most patients who have had RK continue to see a progressive flattening of the cornea resulting in a shift in their refractive error (prescription) from nearsighted to farsighted. Patients who experienced this refractive error shift would go from only needing glasses for distance to now needing them for both distance and near.

Dr. Richard A Driscoll

CHAPTER NINE

The Intra-ocular Lens

The intra-ocular lens is the second most powerful lens of the eye (the cornea is the first), and it is the only adjustable focus lens of the eye.

Cataract Basics

What Are Cataracts?

A cataract is an opacity or cloudiness of the lens inside the eye that causes a reduction in vision.

What Causes Cataracts?

Cataracts may occur as a normal result of aging or secondary to hereditary factors, trauma, inflammation, metabolic, or nutritional disorders, or radiation. Exposure to ultra-violet light can accelerate the formation of certain types of cataracts. Other risk factors for early cataract development include diabetes, smoking, alcohol consumption, steroid use, and poor nutrition.

When Do Cataracts Usually Occur?

On average, you can expect to see cataract formation in your sixties, although this can vary widely. Your eye doctor will be able to examine your eyes for cataract development, so be sure to have your eyes examined annually.

Can I Get Cataracts Again If I Have Surgery?

No, once you have had cataract surgery, your cataracts will not return. When the cataract is removed, the outer layer of the lens (sometimes called the bag) is left in place to hold the new intra-ocular lens implant. After a period of time, usually six months to many years, that outer layer or "bag" turns cloudy, causing patients to think their cataract has returned. It hasn't. The cloudiness can be fixed with an easy in office procedure called a YAG laser capsulotomy.

What Does The Vision Look Like Through A Cataract?

The vision through a cataract would look dim and blurry, with poor contrast. Once a cataract has been removed patients notice that things are not as yellow, but instead they describe the vision as having brighter blues.

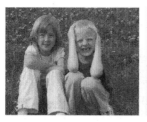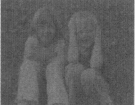

Figure 23   Cataract Vision Simulation

Do They Use A Laser To Take Out A Cataract?

No, not for the initial surgery. When the cataract is removed, part of the intra-ocular lens is left in place to hold the new lens implant. After a while, usually a few years, the membrane that holds the lens implant in place turns cloudy, and a YAG Laser is used to open a window allowing you to once again see clearly. The procedure is simple, painless, and done in the office through dilated pupils.

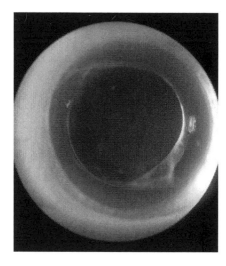

Figure 24   After Cataract Surgery with a Cataract Lens Implant (IOL)

Cataracts Grow Over The Eye, Right?

Cataracts don't grow over the eye. That is called a pterygium (for more information, see page 58). Cataracts are inside the eye and, unless they are quite advanced, someone can't see them just by looking at you.

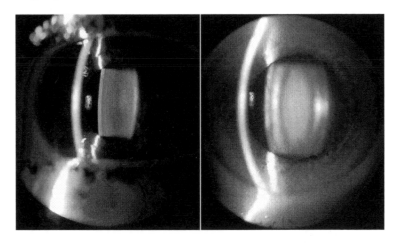

Figure 25   Normal Lens (Left) Nuclear Sclerotic Cataract (Right)

Multifocal Lens Implants

What Can You Tell Me About Those Lens Implants Like The Crystalens?

Bifocal intra-ocular lenses, such as Crystalens, ReZoom, or ReSTOR, give patients some ability to see at near and far, unlike traditional intra-ocular lenses, which only correct for distance vision. The marketing material states that these intra-ocular lenses "fully correct my vision" which can be a little misleading for people thinking that they are going to regain the focusing ability they had when they were thirty.

None of the bifocal intra-ocular lenses available can come close to simulating the focusing ability of the eye. The eye is truly a marvel in how it operates, and it is going to be a while before medical science can duplicate its capabilities. Like bifocal contact lenses, the bifocal IOLs (intra-ocular lens) will reduce your dependency on reading glasses, but they won't make you see like a teenager again.

There are disadvantages to bifocal intra-ocular lenses experienced by some patients, most commonly decreased night vision, poor contrast, and halos. If you are someone who wants the best vision at all distances, then it is probably best to stay with a traditional monofocal intra-ocular lens that will give you good distance vision, then use reading glasses or progressive lenses for near.

Dr. Richard A Driscoll

CHAPTER TEN

Vitreous, Retina, and Optic Nerve

The vitreous occupies the largest part of the eye while the retina and optic nerve translate the light we see into electrical impulses that are then sent to the brain for interpretation. The retina is a sensor, and the optic nerve is like a fiber optic cable that carries data.

Retina

What Is The Retina?

The retina is a light-sensitive tissue at the back of the eye. Its function is similar to that of film in a camera. When light enters the eye, the retina changes the light into nerve signals. The retina then sends these signals along the optic nerve to the brain. Without a retina, the eye cannot communicate with the brain, making vision impossible.

What Is The Macula?

The macula is in the center of the retina. The cornea and the intra-ocular lens focus the light onto your macula, where millions of photoreceptors change the light into nerve signals that show the brain what you are seeing. The macula is where our most acute, sensitive vision is located. Photoreceptors called cones are only found in the macula. They are responsible for our ability to see colors. The cones are densely packed together in the center of the macula, called the fovea, becoming less dense away from the center. There are no cones outside of the macula, thus we don't see colors with our peripheral vision. Conversely, the cones do not see well in the dark. If you want to see something in the dark, don't look directly at it. Look slightly to the side of the object and it will be easier to see.

A Quick Experiment

> In a completely dark room, turn off the TV and cover one eye, look directly at the TV, and it appears dim. Look slightly to the side of the TV and the glowing TV appears much brighter. This is because rods in the retina, which only exist outside the macula, are much more sensitive to light, thus the glowing TV will appear brighter.

Optic Nerve

What Is The Optic Nerve?

The optic nerve is not a true nerve, but an extension of the brain. The optic nerve fibers are bundled together at the optic nerve, and the information we see is taken to the brain to be processed in the visual cortex.

What Is The Blind Spot?

The blind spot is the area of our vision or visual field blocked by our optic nerve. Our blind spot is located about eighteen degrees to the right and below our central vision (point of fixation) in our right eye and to the left and below our central vision in the left eye.

Vitreous

What Is The Vitreous?

The vitreous humor is a fibrous yet clear gel that makes up the back 2/3 of the eye. The primary component of the vitreous humor is hyaluronic acid.

What Are These Black Spots I See?

Floaters are common and can be a scary symptom. "Doctor, I saw dark spots and flashes of light in my eyes and I thought I should come in and have you make sure everything is alright" are words commonly heard by eye doctors and, as a result, flashes and floaters are a common cause of urgent visits to eye doctors' offices.

Flashes and/or floaters can be the signs of serious problems and, as a result, they should always be investigated by your eye doctor. Merely having floaters is not necessarily a problem; it is the recent onset of floaters that requires attention.

How Do Floaters Start?

Floaters occur when a bunch of the fibers that make up the vitreous clump together and cast a shadow on the retina, causing a person to see a black spot or shadow-like image. Patients often describe floaters as looking like a cobweb. Nearsighted people experience floaters more often. Most people have some floaters; however, they are either small enough that they are not bothersome or the brain has learned to ignore them. With the right lighting conditions, almost anyone can see their floaters. Looking up at an overcast sky or a large, lightly colored wall improves one's ability to see their own floaters.

What Is A Posterior Vitreous Detachment?

Floaters also occur when the vitreous humor starts to transition from a gel to a liquid. This liquefacation of the vitreous humor usually occurs later in life. The vitreous starts to liquefy, first from the center, causing the gel to collapse on itself and pull away from the retina, often causing a person to see flashes of light or sparkles, soon to be followed by a bunch of floaters. When the vitreous pulls away from the retina, it is called a posterior vitreous detachment and requires a dilated exam of the retina to verify that the retina was not torn when the vitreous pulled away. Flashes are often the first indication that something is pulling on the retina.

My Floaters Disappeared, What Happened?

With time, gravity allows the floaters to settle below the line of sight, where they will go unnoticed.

I See Something Floating In Front Of Me. What Should I Do?

Most flashes and floaters are harmless; however, all complaints of flashes or floaters of a recent onset require a dilated exam. Occasionally, the pulling on the retina by the vitreous will cause a retinal hole or tear which will ultimately lead to a retinal detachment and permanent vision loss. This type of blindness is almost always preventable by seeking the aid of your eye doctor when you first notice flashes of light or ocular floaters.

Regardless of the patient's age, the recent onset of floaters or flashes should be investigated by an eye doctor with a dilated retinal exam. Your doctor may decide to take retinal photographs as well. Most doctors, when evaluating a patient with floaters, will perform a dilated retinal exam two to three times over the next two months, giving them a reasonable degree of certainty that the vitreous detachment did not cause a retinal hole, tear or detachment.

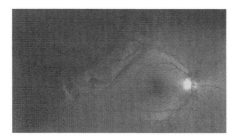

Figure 26   Retinal Detachment

How Do I Get Rid Of My Floaters?

Time is the best medicine for floaters. Surgery is an option, but the potential complications usually make surgery a poor choice. There are no known herbal or natural therapies proven to make your floaters go away. Everyone agrees, floaters are a nuisance, but give them time and they will slowly fade out of sight.

How Long Will My Floaters Last?

The short answer is that your floaters will last between one month and a year or more. I find that the younger you are, the longer it takes for the floaters to go away. As we discussed earlier, the vitreous humor liquefies with age, thus the floaters will go away sooner in an older person because the vitreous is less gelatinous, allowing gravity to do its work and pull the floaters down, out of your line of sight. In a younger person the vitreous humor is much firmer, preventing the floaters from sinking out of sight.

I See Things Float Across My Field Of View

This usually occurs when a person is staring at something and sees a faint, amoeba-like object slowly float across their vision that disappears with a blink. This is caused by debris floating in the tear film.

After Seeing Floaters, What Should I Watch Out For?

This is an important question. When you first saw your floaters, your eye doctor dilated your eyes and told you if you had any retinal holes, tears, or retinal detachments. Typically, when we are following a patient with a recent onset of floaters, we want to dilate our patient's eyes a few times over the next sixty days to see if the vitreous pulling away from your retina causes a retinal hole, tear, or detachment. If at any time between visits, or at any time for that matter, you notice an increase in the size or number of floaters, flashes of light, or if you see a curtain appear in your peripheral vision from any direction top, bottom, left, or right, you should call your eye doctor. Chances are that your eye doctor will want to dilate your eyes again.

The recurrence of flashes or floaters doesn't necessarily mean that your posterior vitreous detachment has caused a retinal hole, tear, or a detachment. More than likely it means that the vitreous humor is continuing to pull on your retina. The only way to know if this change in presentation is serious is to see your doctor and have your eyes dilated again.

Why Do You Push On My Eye With That Thing When My Eyes Are Dilated?

That "thing" is a sceral depressor, used to help us get a better look at retinal holes and tears in the periphery of the retina.

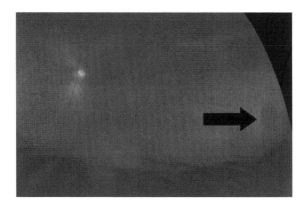

Figure 27   Retinal Hole via Optomap

Macular Degeneration

What Is Macular Degeneration?

Age-related macular degeneration (AMD) is a disease that affects your central vision. It is a common cause of vision loss among people over age of sixties. As a matter of fact, it is the leading cause of blindness for people over age 55 in the US. Approximately 1.5% of the US population over age forty has a form of macular degeneration. The incidence increases with age.[22] Because only the center of your vision is usually affected, people do not go totally blind from macular degeneration. However, AMD can sometimes make it difficult to read, drive, or perform other daily activities that require fine, central vision.

I Heard There Are Two Types Of AMD, What Are They?

There are two forms of macular degeneration, the wet form and the dry form.

What Is Dry AMD?

Dry AMD is the most common type of macular degeneration, accounting for about 90% of all cases. There is no treatment for Dry AMD, however patients with dry AMD experience much less vision loss than patients with wet AMD. The cause of dry AMD is unknown.

What is Wet AMD?

Wet AMD gets its name from the fact that the vision loss is due retinal damage caused by leaking blood vessels under the retina. Although only 10% of all people with AMD have wet AMD, it accounts for 90% of the vision loss from macular degeneration. The wet form of macular degeneration almost always progresses at a much faster rate than the dry form of AMD.

How Does Dry AMD Damage Vision?

Photoreceptors are the light sensitive cells in the retina that slowly degenerate. As these photoreceptors break down, the central vision is affected with a decrease in visual acuity. Dry AMD often occurs in just one eye at first. Dry macular degeneration may occur in the other eye, however it may not necessarily be to the same degree. There is no way to predict if or when both eyes will be affected.

How Does Wet AMD Damage Vision?

With the wet form of macular degeneration, blood vessels begin to grow under the macula. These new blood vessels are fragile, thus easily prone to leaking. When the blood vessels leak, they cause the macula to become distorted. An early symptom of wet AMD is a slight distortion in vision. The blood vessels may stop leaking in which case the vision levels off and a small scar usually develops. The lesion may leak again at a later time, causing greater distortion, decreased vision, and a larger scar.

What Are Drusen?

Drusen are small, yellow deposits located in or around the macula. The presence of a few drusen does not mean a person has macular degeneration; however, eyes that have drusen present are at a greater risk for AMD-related vision loss. Drusen can be present while the vision is unaffected; however, a lot of drusen clustered together in the center of the macula will typically cause a reduction in visual acuity.

Who Is At Risk For AMD?

Although AMD can occur during middle age, the risk of AMD increases greatly as we age. Results of a large study showed that people in their fifties have about a two percent chance of getting AMD. This risk rises to nearly 30% in those between age 75 to 85. Besides age, other AMD risk factors include:

Smoking

Smoking at least doubles your risk of AMD.[23] Also smokers should not take supplements recommended to prevent AMD containing beta carotene as this appears to increase their risk for lung cancer.

Family History

People with a family history of AMD appear to be at a greater risk. Having a first degree relative (parents, siblings, or offspring) with AMD increases your risk by 2.4 times.[24]

Cholesterol

People with elevated levels of blood cholesterol are at a higher risk for early AMD.[25]

Obesity

There are conflicting studies here; however, one of the most recent studies indicated that there was a 13% increase in the odds of early AMD in men for each 0.1 inch increase in the waist/hip ratio. However, the study did not show the same results for women.[26] The preponderance of scientific evidence indicates that poor diet/nutrition are linked to AMD.

What Are The Symptoms Of AMD?

Neither dry nor wet AMD causes any pain. The most common symptom of dry AMD is slightly blurred vision. You may need more light for reading or other tasks. Also, you may find it hard to recognize faces until you are close to them.

The picture below on the left shows how a normal person would view the scene. The photos in the middle and to the right simulate how a person affected with macular degeneration might view the scene. If you notice any of these changes in your vision, call your eye doctor at once for an eye exam.

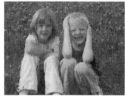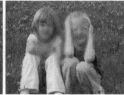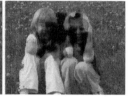

Figure 28   Macular Degeneration Simulation

What Are the Symptoms Of Dry AMD?

As dry AMD gets worse, you may see a blurred spot in the center of your vision. This spot occurs because a group of cells (photoreceptors) in the macula have stopped working properly. Over time, the blurred spot may get bigger and darker, taking more of your central vision.

People with dry AMD in one eye often do not notice any changes in their vision. With one eye seeing clearly, they can still drive, read, and see fine details. Some people may notice changes in their vision only if AMD affects both eyes. It is quite difficult for a patients to notice that they have dry AMD since many other, more common conditions also cause blurred vision, thus making early detection with regular eye exams very important.

What Are the Symptoms Of Wet AMD?

An early symptom of wet AMD is that straight lines appear wavy or distorted. This distortion, called metamorphopsia, occurs when newly formed blood vessels leak fluid under the macula. This fluid raises the macula and distorts your vision. Another sign that you may have wet AMD is rapid loss of your central vision. This is different from dry AMD in which loss of central vision occurs slowly. As in dry AMD, you may also notice a blind spot in or near your central vision.

Can I Eat Certain Foods To Prevent The Progression Of AMD?

Contrary to popular belief, carrots are not the best food for our eyes. Dark leafy green vegetables such as spinach are better for our eyes because they contain a higher concentration of lutein and zeaxanthin.

Will A Healthy Lifestyle Offer Protection Against AMD?

A recent study of women evaluated the eating habits, amount of exercise, and smoking history. The women who scored in the top 20% for those factors lowered their risk of early AMD by three-fold when compared to the women in the bottom 20%.[27] So, yes, it appears that a healthy lifestyle does lower your risk for AMD.

I Heard Lutein And Zeaxanthin Are Good For My Eyes, How Much Should I Take?

Current studies recommend 10 mg of lutein and 2 mg of zeaxanthin per day as a preventative for macular degeneration.

Does Cataract Surgery Increase The Risk Of Macular Degeneration?

This is a question with a degree of conflicting research which I will sort out for you here. Some of the most recent research in a 2009 study of 108 patients indicated that cataract surgery did not increase the incidence of macular degeneration.[28] What some of the earlier, conflicting studies did not take into account was that, by removing the cataract, it made it easier to identify early cases of macular degeneration masked by the cataract. Following cataract surgery, an eye doctor can better visualize the fundus, and the patient becomes more aware of subtle vision changes. All of these things allow for earlier diagnosis of macular degeneration.

So there is not a clear link between cataract surgery and macular degeneration. My impression is that cataract surgery is not a cause of macular degeneration, but merely allows for improved detection.

How Is AMD Detected?

We detect AMD during an eye examination. A comprehensive eye exam will typically include more tests than what is shown below; however, it should include at least the following tests:

Visual Acuity
Called the Snellen Eye Chart, it measures how well you see at distance or "optical infinity."

Refraction
A refraction is helpful in determining what your best vision would be when you are wearing the right eyeglasses. Often patients present with old glasses that are not allowing them to see their best. A refraction helps the doctor rule out a simple cause of decreased vision, such as myopia or hyperopia.

Pupil Dilation/Fundus Exam
This examination enables us to see more of the retina and look for signs of AMD. To do this, drops are placed into your eye to dilate (widen) the pupil. Once your eyes are dilated, your doctor will shine bright lights in your eyes that will allow the back of your eye

(your fundus or retina) to be viewed. After the examination, your vision may remain blurred, and you may be sensitive to bright light for several hours.

One of the most common early signs of AMD is the presence of drusen. Drusen are tiny yellow deposits in the retina. We can see them during an eye examination. The presence of drusen alone does not indicate macular degeneration, but it might mean that the eye is at risk for developing more severe AMD.

Amsler Grid

While conducting the examination, your eye doctor may ask you to look at an Amsler grid. This grid is a pattern that resembles a checkerboard or piece of graph paper. You will be asked to cover one eye and stare at a black dot in the center of the grid. While staring at the dot, you may notice that the straight lines in the pattern appear wavy, distorted, or missing. (See Amsler Grid below.)

Below is a normal Amsler grid:

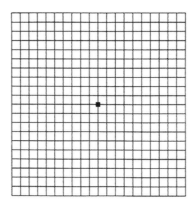

Figure 29   Normal Amsler Grid

These grids are reduced in size. To monitor your vision, use the Amsler Grid later in this section.

The Amsler Grid for a person experiencing metamorphopsia from macular degeneration would look something like this.

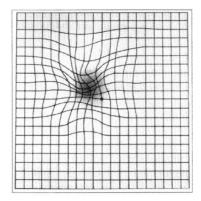

Figure 30   Distorted Amsler Grid

Additional Testing

Your doctor may suggest additional tests, such as photographs of your retina, OCT (optical coherence tomographer), or fluorescein angiography.

Fundus Photos

We have all heard that a picture is worth a thousand words. In medicine it is no different. Photography is important part of modern medicine. Photographs are essential in allowing us to document what your retina looks like now, giving us a reference point to notice subtle changes over time.

OCT

Optical Coherence Tomography (OCT) is one of the newest technologies available to us. The OCT uses a scanning laser to make hundreds of near infra-red laser scans and puts them together to make a three dimensional picture of your retina or optic nerve. It also uses a database of scans from "normal" people to see if your data falls within the expected range. Good scans can usually be obtained without pupil dilation, though larger pupils does make it easier. Most of the newer OCTs have software that compares a patient's prior scans, looking for subtle, early retinal changes, thus further improving early detection of macular degeneration.

Fluorescein Angiography

A special dye is injected into a vein in your arm and a series of pictures are then taken as the dye passes through the retinal blood vessels. Your doctor will then look at the series of photos to see if any of the blood vessels are leaking. With these photos he/she will then be able to determine if treatment is necessary and, if so, what type.

How Is AMD Treated?

There is no cure for dry AMD or wet AMD. This does not mean however that you will lose your sight and become completely blind. There are treatments available.

Treating Dry AMD

Fortunately, dry AMD progresses slowly. You may notice a gradual decrease in your central vision over the years. In many patients the vision will stabilize with no decline in vision. The vast majority of patients with dry AMD are able to lead normal, active lives. Studies have shown prevention, with antioxidant therapy, reduces the chances and rate of the progression of AMD. All patients with dry AMD should monitor their vision daily with an Amsler Grid. A change in the grid could signal that the dry AMD is converting to wet AMD. This does not happen frequently; however, should it happen, it is important to detect and treat this as soon as possible.

Finally, don't skip your regular eye exams. Your eye doctor will discuss with you how often he/she wants to see you. Regular eye exams are important since it is often difficult for a patient to detect subtle macular degeneration changes. In the eye, it is much easier to prevent a problem than to fix it; thus, early detection is important.

Treating Wet AMD

Baby Boomers are now entering the age where macular degeneration is much more common. This has driven research into treatment and preventative therapies. None of the current therapies will restore lost vision. They are all aimed at treating the current condition to prevent further vision loss, thus frequent monitoring is important.

Laser Surgery

Once the mainstay of macular degeneration treatment, laser surgery involved focusing a high energy laser beam onto the small, new leaking blood vessels. The laser would cause a small scar, destroying the blood vessels. Unfortunately, the laser would also destroy some of the surrounding normal retinal tissue and, often with it, a further reduction in vision. A small loss in additional vision was deemed necessary to prevent a rapid and usually greater loss of vision should the lesion be left untreated. Laser surgery is still used today; however, with less invasive options available, it is left for lesions that are not near the central vision. Laser surgery will not prevent new blood vessels from forming or leaking. Laser surgery treats the blood vessels currently present and additional treatments may be needed.

Photodynamic Therapy

A relatively non invasive treatment, photodynamic therapy involves injecting a drug called Verteporfin (trade name Visudyne) into the arm. The drug sticks to abnormal blood vessels and is usually used to treat blood vessels directly under the fovea. Once the drug has been allowed to circulate, a special light is shined into the eye. The drug then destroys the abnormal blood vessels. Most patients receiving photodynamic therapy (PDT) will have multiple treatment sessions. Following PDT treatment, it is recommended that patients avoid bright indoor and outdoor lights for five days.

Anti-VEGF Injections

The Anti-VEGF injections are the newest treatment for wet AMD. There are three Anti-VEGF medications, Ranibizumab (Lucentis), and Pegaptanib Sodium (Macugen) are FDA approved for the treatment of wet AMD. Bevacizumab (Avastin) is an anti cancer medication, similar to Lucentis, that has also been found effective in the treatment of wet AMD, though it is not FDA approved for this use.

In the past few years the anti-VEGF (Vascular Endothelial Growth Factor) medications have been found to be the most successful treatment for wet macular degeneration.

Which Is Better In The Treatment Of Wet AMD Avastin Or Lucentis?

Two recent studies showed that both medications were equally effective in the treatment of macular degeneration; however, patients receiving Avastin had a slightly higher rate of serious systemic complications requiring hospitalization.[29] The authors concluded that the higher complication rate required further study and could not be directly attributed to the medications.[30]

Which Is Better, Anti VEGF Or PDT Treatment?

Both treatments are an important part of wet AMD therapy, and this is a subject to discuss in detail with your retinal specialist. Good studies have directly compared Visudyne PDT and Lucentis and found that, while both therapies were effective overall, Lucentis provided better results during the two year study period.[31]

What Research Is Being Done?

The National Eye Institute (NEI) is the Federal government's lead agency for vision research. The NEI is supporting a number of research studies both in the laboratory and with patients to learn more about the cause of AMD. This research should provide better ways to detect, treat, and prevent vision loss in people with the disease.

Findings from the NEI-sponsored Age-related Eye Disease Study (AREDS) showed that high levels of antioxidants and zinc significantly reduced the risk of advanced age-related macular degeneration (AMD) by about 25 percent.

Scientists have begun to study the possibility of transplanting healthy cells into a diseased retina. Although this work is at an early stage and still experimental, someday it may help people keep their vision or restore some lost vision.

What Can You Do To Protect Your Vision From AMD?

Protecting Your Eyes From Dry AMD

If you have dry AMD, you should have your eyes examined through dilated pupils at least once a year. Regular eye exams will allow your eye doctor to monitor your condition and evaluate you for other conditions as well.

Your eye doctor will probably provide you with an Amsler Grid and instructions for use at home. The Amsler Grid provides you with a quick, inexpensive way to evaluate your vision each day for signs of progression to wet AMD. You also may want to check your vision by reading the newspaper, watching television, and just looking at people's faces. If you detect any changes, you should call your eye doctor immediately.

As discussed earlier antioxidant supplements have been shown to be effective in preventing early dry AMD from progressing to wet AMD. Quitting smoking will also improve your odds of keeping your vision, as was found in the Blue Mountains Eye Study.

Protecting Your Eyes From Wet AMD

If you have wet AMD, it is important not to delay procedures recommended by your eye doctor. After surgery, you will need to have frequent eye examinations to detect any recurrence of leaking blood vessels. And, of course, stop smoking. Studies have shown that people who smoke have a greater risk of recurrence of leaking blood vessels than those who don't.

In addition, you should continue to check your vision (at home with the Amsler Grid or other methods) as described under dry AMD, and schedule an eye exam immediately if you detect any changes.

Where Can I Find An Amsler Grid To Monitor My AMD?

We have included one here. Feel free to tear it out and place it on your refrigerator or some other prominent place where you will see it every day. To use the Amsler Grid, place it twelve inches from your eye. While covering one eye at a time, look through the bifocal of your glasses focusing on the dot in the center. When looking at the center dot, using your peripheral vision, you should see all four corners. The lines should be straight, not wavy or missing. If you notice any distortion in the grid pattern, you should call your eye doctor right away. The Amsler Grid is best used to monitor your macular degeneration between doctor visits.

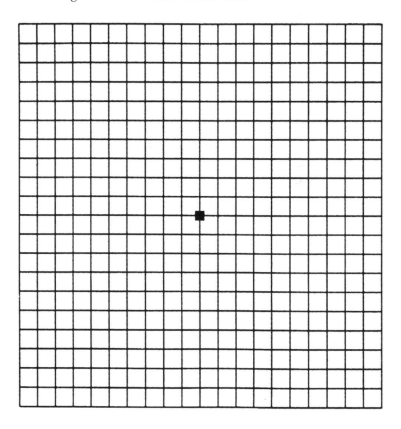

Figure 31   Amsler Grid

This page is left blank so you can tear out the Amsler Grid page and place it somewhere that you will see it daily.

What Can You Do If You Have Already Lost Vision To AMD?

Normal use of your eyes will not cause further damage to your vision. Even if you have lost sight to AMD, you should not be afraid to use your eyes for reading, watching TV, and other activities.

Low vision aids are available to help you make the most of your remaining vision. Low vision aids are special lenses or electronic systems that make images appear larger.

If you find that your vision loss is having a detrimental impact on your ability to complete everyday tasks, discuss this with your eye doctor as he can make suggestions and recommend other professionals who can help maximize the vision that you do have. In addition, organizations and agencies offer information about counseling, training, and other special services available.

I Heard Taking Aspirin Will Cause Wet Macular Degeneration

The study referenced in this question was published online right before this book was about to go to press. This European study stated that patients with wet AMD who were taking daily aspirin appeared to progress at a faster rate than wet AMD patients who were not taking aspirin.[32] The study did not conclude that taking aspirin daily caused the wet AMD; however, it did appear that aspirin may have made wet AMD progress at a faster rate. Further studies into this question clearly need to be done.

Glaucoma: An Overview

Certainly questions about glaucoma are among the most commonly asked of eye doctors. However, "what is glaucoma" has to be in the top five of questions most asked of eye doctors.

What Is Glaucoma?

In basic terms, glaucoma is a progressive disease of the optic nerve caused when the pressure inside the eye is higher than the optic nerve can withstand. The most common form of glaucoma will cause a patient to slowly lose vision. The peripheral vision is usually affected first; however, when glaucoma affects a younger person it has often been noted that a loss in central vision precedes a peripheral vision loss. Without proper testing, this decreased vision will go unnoticed by a patient for many years. Left untreated, glaucoma will ultimately result in blindness.

Who Is At Risk For Glaucoma?

Although anyone can get glaucoma, some people are at higher risk than others. Some of the most common risk factors include:

- Being of African American race
- Over age forty
- People with a family history of glaucoma
- Patients with diabetes

What Are My Chances Of Getting Glaucoma?

Almost 2.0% of Americans have been diagnosed with glaucoma. Approximately one fourth of those diagnosed with glaucoma are African Americans. Worldwide, 2.4 million people per year are diagnosed with glaucoma. African Americans are three times more likely to have been diagnosed with glaucoma. The prevalence of glaucoma increases with age. By the year 2020 it is estimated that the number of patients diagnosed with glaucoma in the United States will increase by 50% to 3.6 million patients. Glaucoma accounts for approximately 12% of all new cases of legal blindness each year. It has been estimated that only one half of the patients with glaucoma have been diagnosed. [33]

What Role Does Age Play In Developing Glaucoma?

The risk of developing glaucoma increases with age; however, children and babies can also have glaucoma. As a general rule, the risk for glaucoma doubles for every ten years of age. There are twice as many seventy-year-old patients with glaucoma as there are sixty-year-old patients with glaucoma.

Is There A Gene That Causes Glaucoma?

Research funded by Fort Worth-based Alcon has found that the over expression of the gene sFRP1 elevates the pressure in an eye, thus greatly increasing a patient's risk for developing glaucoma. Discovery of a gene responsible for causing glaucoma is great news. Glaucoma is the second leading cause of irreversible blindness in the United States. Making the diagnosis of glaucoma at its early stage is often difficult. Early diagnosis is important to prevent loss of a patient's peripheral vision. New technology, such as scanning laser ophthalmoscopes, have made early diagnosis much more reliable; however, a gene test would be great. I hope we will be able to use this technology in our offices soon.

What Is The Optic Nerve's Function?

The optic nerve is like a cable made up of over one million nerve fibers that carry the information collected by your eye (retina) to the visual cortex of the brain for processing. Glaucoma slowly decreases the ability of your optic nerve to carry this information to your brain.

Why Does Glaucoma Cause A Loss Of Vision?

The build up of pressure in your eye causes glaucoma by damaging the optic nerve or retinal nerve fibers. Attachments to the ciliary body, a small muscle that actually helps our eye change focus, also produces a fluid called aqueous humor in your eye. The pressure increases in the eye because aqueous humor is being produced too quickly or it is not being drained from the eye fast enough. The production and drainage systems must be balanced or the pressure will build up, causing glaucomatous damage to the optic nerve.

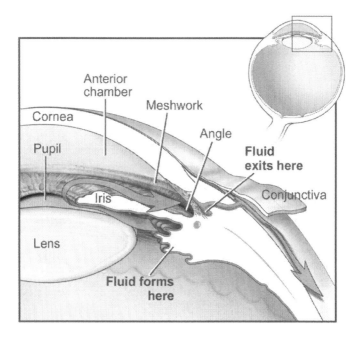

Figure 32   Intra-ocular Fluid Dynamics

There are currently two basic theories as to why excessive ocular pressure causes glaucoma.

1. **The Vascular Theory** High intra-ocular pressure decreases blood flow to the optic nerve.

2. **The Physical Theory** The high pressure, over time, physically crushes and kills the individual nerve fibers.

Interestingly, some cutting edge research out of Vanderbilt University by David Calkins, Ph.D. was published in the *Proceedings of the National Academy of Sciences*. Dr. Calkins hypothesizes that glaucoma first starts in the brain like other central nervous system disorders, with the ocular signs being a late manifestation.[34] Currently, Dr. Calkins' research is directed toward looking for medical therapies that can restore the connection of the nerve fibers between the brain and the retina. The optic nerve is not a true nerve. It is really an extension of the brain, thus Dr. Calkins' theory, if proven to be true, will revolutionize the way we diagnose and treat glaucoma.

Another current thought on glaucoma is that patients with a lower cerebral spinal fluid pressure are more susceptible to the high pressure in the eye, and this may be the cause of low tension glaucoma.

What Are The Symptoms Of Glaucoma?

At first, open-angle glaucoma has no symptoms. Vision stays normal, and there is no pain. If glaucoma remains untreated, central vision will initially remain unaffected. However, with time, objects will begin to be missed to the side or out of the corner of the eye, and with time, an increased difficulty seeing at night. Typically, patients will notice no symptoms related to glaucoma until the late stages of the condition. This is why glaucoma has been called "the sneak thief of sight."

What Happens If Glaucoma Is Left Untreated?

Without treatment, patients with glaucoma will find that they eventually have no side or peripheral vision. It may seem as though they are looking through a tunnel. Over time, the remaining central vision may decrease until there is no vision left. Optic nerve damage caused by glaucoma is permanent; therefore, it is important to seek treatment in the early stages of the disease rather than waiting until symptoms are noticed.

What Would My Vision Look Like If I Had Glaucoma?

In the early to moderate stages of glaucoma you probably won't notice any changes. However, in the advanced stages of glaucoma, you may notice a decrease in your peripheral vision and poor night vision. As the glaucoma progresses, the central island of good vision will continue to contract. With early detection, modern medications, laser treatment, and surgical management, the number of patients going blind from glaucoma is low.

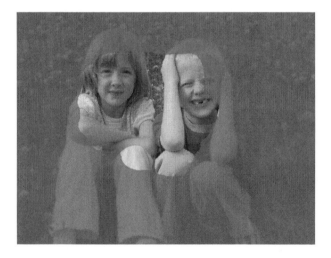

Figure 33   Simulating Moderate Vision Loss in Glaucoma

Does Glaucoma Always Affect The Peripheral Vision First?

No, not always. Most of the time the peripheral vision is the first to be affected. However, often in younger patients with glaucoma, a visual field defect will develop initially near their central vision, with an early symptom being a decrease in central visual acuity.

My Pressure is 25. I Have Glaucoma, Right?

Most people think that they have glaucoma if the pressure in their eye is high. This is not always true. Yes, high pressure puts you at a greater risk for glaucoma; however, an elevated pressure by itself does not make the diagnosis of glaucoma.

Whether or not you get glaucoma depends on the level of pressure that your optic nerve can tolerate without being damaged. This level is different for each person. Although normal pressure is usually said to be between 12-21 mm Hg, a person might have glaucoma even if the pressure is in this range. Conversely, having a pressure over 21 does not mean a person has glaucoma. This is why an eye examination and appropriate testing are important.

Many factors are considered when making the diagnosis of glaucoma. The intra-ocular pressure is just a small part of the deciding factors. The appearance of the optic nerve, the family/medical history, visual fields, and scanning laser ophthalmoscopy are much more important than the intra-ocular pressure in making the initial diagnosis of glaucoma. Once the diagnosis is made, however, the pressure becomes an important indicator in evaluating the effectiveness of the treatment.

What Tests Are Used To Diagnose Glaucoma?

Traditionally glaucoma was diagnosed by evaluating a patient's peripheral vision with a visual field. Recent advances in laser technology, along with new studies, have improved our ability to diagnose glaucoma more accurately and at an earlier stage. A patient being evaluated for glaucoma will typically have the following tests.

What Is A Comprehensive, Dilated Eye Exam?

Diagnosing glaucoma starts with an eye exam. The eye exam should include a complete review of your medications and your personal and family medical histories. An initial ocular health evaluation will also be completed, typically through dilated pupils. Some of the additional testing noted below also requires dilation; therefore, your doctor may need to dilate you a second time. For more information on what makes a complete eye exam, see page 167.

What Is Gonioscopy?

A lens is placed on the eye that lets the doctor evaluate the trabecular meshwork. The trabecular meshwork is located where the cornea, sclera, and iris meet. The trabecular meshwork allows the fluid in the eye to drain into our lymphatic system.

What is Tonometry?

Tonometry is how we measure the pressure in the eye. There are numerous ways to do this. The most common is with a Goldmann tonometer. Anesthetic eye drops with a dye are placed in the patient's eyes, and a blue light is then directed onto the tonometer tip. The tonometer tip measures the cornea by lightly applanating the patient's cornea.

What Is Pachymetry?

Pachymetry involves measuring the thickness of the cornea. One of the major findings of the Ocular Hypertension Treatment Study was that if we were measuring the internal pressure of the eye through a thick cornea, the pressure would measure falsely high. Conversely, if the cornea is thin, the pressure will be measured lower than the actual pressure.[35] Therefore, to know the true intra-ocular pressure, we measure the cornea's thickness.

What Are Fundus Photos?

The retinal fundus is the back of the eye or retina. Pictures of the eye are helpful to look for changes in the appearance of the optic nerve over time. Fundus photos can be done dilated or undilated, depending on the type of retinal camera.

What Is The Threshold Visual Field?

Since the primary symptom of glaucoma is a progressive decrease in peripheral vision, one of the most important tests to evaluate our peripheral vision is a visual field. In the simplest terms, a visual field detects how dim of a light can be seen in the patient's peripheral vision. The brighter the light needs to be before a patient reports seeing it, the more advanced the glaucoma.

Most visual used in the diagnosis of glaucoma are completed through dilated pupils. Visual fields are always done one eye at a time. During the visual field, the patient looks straight ahead at a small fixation light and presses a handheld button when she sees a small, round light flash in her peripheral vision. Some of the flashes will be bright, some of them dim and barely noticeable. Visual Fields are typically repeated every six to twelve months.

What Is A Scanning Laser Ophthalmoscope?

The most recent advancement in the detection and diagnosis of glaucoma is the scanning laser ophthalmoscope. There are numerous types of scanning laser ophthalmoscopes (SLO). The SLO can be used to measure the thickness of the various layers of the retina, to make a topographical map of the optic nerve or to take a retinal photograph.

How Does The Scanning Laser Ophthalmoscope Work?

The SLO takes a series of retinal scans using an infra-red laser (usually from 16 to over 500 depending on the model and the intended use). Using computer software, the SLO puts the scans together to make a three dimensional image or panoramic photo much like an MRI. In the treatment of glaucoma the SLO allows us to see damage caused by glaucoma before the patient experiences a loss of peripheral vision.

How Is The Scanning Laser Used To Diagnose And Treat Glaucoma?

The SLO measures the thickness of the nerve fibers leading into the optic nerve. Retinal nerve fibers are like wires that carry the information of what you see from the photo receptors to the optic nerve, then ultimately to the visual cortex where the brain translates this information into an image for us to see. In glaucoma, these nerve fibers become damaged and die. The SLO measures how thick the nerve fibers are that lead into the optic nerve. As nerve fibers die off, the nerve fiber layer thins out. The SLO not only allows the doctor to compare changes in the nerve fiber thickness over time, but it also compares the data to the expected range for "normal" patients who do not have glaucoma.

How Is Glaucoma Treated?

Glaucoma is a life-long condition that will always require treatment, much like hypertension and diabetes. We can control these diseases; however, we cannot, as of yet, cure them. Today there are numerous ophthalmic medications available to us in the treatment of glaucoma. Some are eye drops used only once a day; others are used up to four times a day. More than one medication may be used to treat glaucoma. If glaucoma cannot be controlled with medications, other procedures, including surgery, may be considered.

The concern of most patients is will I go blind from glaucoma? That is difficult to answer and depends on numerous factors. Due to the many excellent medications available today, most people, with early treatment, will not go blind from glaucoma. The rate of blindness from glaucoma is much lower today than ever before. Early detection is the key.

What Can I Do To Decrease My Chances Of Going Blind?

Glaucomatous blindness is preventable with the current available treatments. Using the medications as prescribed and seeking regularly scheduled office visits are crucial to preventing the progression of glaucoma. It is best to monitor the pressure three to four times per year, repeat visual fields at least annually, and take photographs of the optic nerve every one to two years. Some of these office visits will be a brief check of the intra-ocular pressure, whereas others may include your annual eye exam, visual fields, photos of your optic nerves, or imaging of your optic nerve with a scanning laser ophthalmoscope.

You can also help protect the vision of family members and friends who may be at high risk for glaucoma, especially African Americans over age forty and everyone over age sixty. Encourage your family members at risk for glaucoma to have an eye examination every year.

What Is The Best Way To Take Eye Drops?

If you forget your drops one day, don't try to make it up on the next day. Try to be relatively consistent with the time of day you use your drops. If you are late taking your drop, it's best not to skip that dosing altogether; just move up your time schedule for that day, then resume your normal schedule the next morning. Taking more drops than prescribed will not make your pressure any lower. Only take your drops the prescribed number of times per day. On the day of your appointment, remember to take your drops as you normally do.

If you happen to forget to take your drops on the day of your office visit, please tell your doctor. He or she will appreciate knowing how consistent you are with your eye drop schedule. Being honest with your doctor about your drop schedule will prevent an incorrect conclusion that the reason your pressure is high is because your current medication regimen is no longer working, rather than the correct conclusion that your pressure may be high because you forgot your drops.

Often, patients are taken aback when they first learn that they have glaucoma or that they are at an increased risk. Your doctor's job is to educate you; therefore, no question is too small. Your eye doctor should have no problem answering questions. Doctors want their patients to be well informed about their condition. Answering questions is a part of what we must do.

If My Blood Pressure Is High Does That Mean The Pressure In My Eye Is High, Too?

This is a great question that gets asked a lot. The pressure inside your eye is completely unrelated to your blood pressure. The intra-ocular pressure system and blood pressure are completely separate systems, and fluid is not exchanged between them. Therefore, if you have high blood pressure, you won't necessarily have glaucoma.

Facts About Glaucoma

Is Glaucoma More Common In African Americans Than In Caucasians?

Glaucoma is three to five times more common in African Americans than Caucasians. While glaucoma is the third most common cause of blindness in Caucasian Americans, it is the most common cause of blindness in African Americans.

Does Glaucoma Tend To Run In Families?

Having a family history of glaucoma does not guarantee that one's descendants will also have glaucoma; however, it does markedly increase their chances for developing glaucoma. A comprehensive, dilated eye exam is recommended every one to two years for anyone who has an immediate family member with a history of glaucoma.

Can I Tell If I Have Glaucoma?

In the early to middle stages of open angle glaucoma, there are no symptoms that a patient could observe. The early stages of open-angle glaucoma, the most common form, usually have no warning signs. However, in the later stages of glaucoma, a patients may notice that the peripheral vision is not clear and the night vision has gotten worse.

Does Glaucoma Hurt?

No, open angle glaucoma, by far the most common form, is painless. Narrow angle glaucoma, on the other hand, is associated with acute ocular and head pain, nausea, redness, and an abrupt decrease in vision.

Is There A Cure For Glaucoma?

Although glaucoma cannot be cured, it can usually be controlled with eye drops, conventional surgery, or laser surgery. Sometimes eye doctors will recommend a combination of surgery and medication to control the intra ocular pressure.

What Causes Glaucoma?

In its simplest terms, glaucoma is caused by pressure inside the eye greater than the optic nerve and the retinal nerve fibers can tolerate, resulting in a loss of peripheral vision. A high intra ocular pressure alone, however, does not mean a person has glaucoma. There are numerous factors that contribute to the diagnosis of glaucoma. Some new theories, however suggest glaucoma may first occur in the brain and that the ocular damage is merely a later manifestation of the condition.

Can Glaucoma Damage Be Reversed?

No, vision loss from glaucoma is permanent. However, with the new treatments available, most patients can be successfully treated, preserving their vision.

Will The "Glaucoma Test" Tell Me If I Have Glaucoma?

Tonometry, often referred to as "the puff test," is often thought, by patients, to be the glaucoma test. The pressure as measured in the eye, though helpful in making the diagnosis of glaucoma, is really only part of the entire process. By itself, the intra-ocular pressure measurement is not an accurate or reliable "glaucoma detector."

A doctor most often becomes suspicious of glaucoma while performing a routine eye exam. The diagnosis of glaucoma, however, is made through interpretation of additional diagnostic tests, such as visual fields, optic nerve photographs, optical coherence tomography, pachymetry, gonioscopy, and a dilated fundus exam. A patient's family and personal medical history are also evaluated.

Should People At Risk For Glaucoma Have An Eye Examination Through Dilated Pupils?

Some of the diagnostic testing must be done through undilated pupils; however, visual fields are most often conducted through dilated pupils. A dilated fundus exam is also important in diagnosing glaucoma because it gives the doctor a stereoscopic or 3D view of the optic nerve.

I Heard You Can Smoke Marijuana For Glaucoma?

Well, kind of . . . "Mary Jane" does lower the pressure in the eye when smoked; however, its affect doesn't last long. You would have to smoke about eight joints a day to lower your eye pressure. Even if you could smoke enough marijuana, the pressure lowering effect of marijuana is not as effective as current glaucoma medications. Incorporating the active ingredient of marijuana into an eye drop has been studied and found to be ineffective.[36]

Now, I've not partaken in this mode of therapy before, nor have I ever prescribed it for a patient, but I think it would be rather difficult to get much done if you are constantly smoking a joint or trying to pacify your munchies.

The optomap® Retinal Exam

What Is The optomap® Retinal Exam?

The **opto**map® Retinal Exam is a scanning laser ophthalmoscope that provides a panoramic view of the back of a person's eye (the retina). The **opto**map® allows your doctor to view over 80% of the retina without dilating the pupils.

How Does The *optomap*® Work?

The **opto**map® uses two scanning lasers to take sixteen digital pictures of the back of the eye in about one fourth of a second. The computer then merges those pictures into a single panoramic photograph.

The patient places the eye to be photographed up to the instrument, and the doctor's assistant positions the patient for a photograph and takes the picture. The photographer will take two photographs of your eye and, if the image quality, is good repeat the process on the other eye.

Why Is The *optomap*® Better Than Dilation?

The **opto**map® is not necessarily better than pupillary dilation. The **opto**map® Retinal Exam is a great tool to use in addition to dilation or when a patient can't, or doesn't want to, be dilated.

In some cases the view provided by the **opto**map® is superior to that afforded by pupil dilation. For example, a patient who is light sensitive will often refuse to have her pupils dilated because of the pain she experience while being examined. The dilated view of a photosensitive patient's fundus is often poor because it is difficult for the patient to keep her eyes open or to look in the appropriate direction. The **opto**map® captures an image with a brief flash that even light sensitive patients do not object to, allowing the doctor to view the ocular fundus without discomfort to the patient. The **opto**map® allows for a more comfortable retinal exam.

A dilated fundus exam, on the other hand, provides the doctor with a three dimensional or stereoscopic view as well as allowing the doctor to view almost 100% of the retina. The best option would be to have both, as they each have a lot to offer in providing a more comprehensive eye exam.

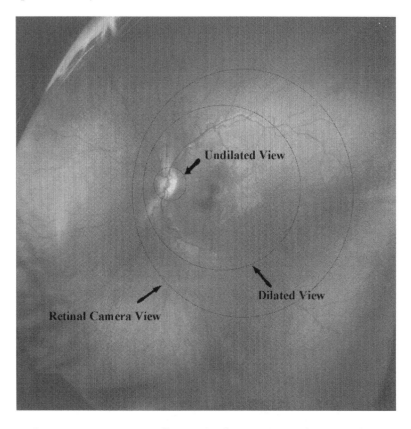

Figure 34   Comparing Different Fundus Viewing Techniques

The image above is from the **opto**map® Retinal Camera comparing the doctor's view of your eye through an undilated pupil with an instrument called a direct ophthalmoscope (inner ring). The second largest ring is the view as seen through dilated pupils with an instrument worn on the head called a binocular indirect ophthalmoscope (BIO). The BIO will allow the doctor to see almost 100% of the retina if the patient looks in multiple directions while the doctor readjusts his or her light. The third ring is the view from a good retinal camera.

For Whom Is The *opto*map® Recommended?

The short answer is almost everyone is a good candidate for the **opto**map® Retinal Exam. We find, however, that some of the best candidates for the **opto**map® Retinal Exam are those patients who can't or don't want to be dilated, children, anyone with a history of eye problems such as diabetic retinopathy, glaucoma, and people who are light sensitive, just to name a few.

What You Want To Know About Diabetic Retinopathy

Diabetic retinopathy is a potentially blinding complication of diabetes that damages the retina of the eye. Diabetic retinopathy eventually affects nearly half of all Americans diagnosed with diabetes. Approximately 3.4% of the US population has some form of diabetic retinopathy.[37]

Will I Know If I Have Diabetic Retinopathy?

At first, you may notice no changes in your vision. But don't let diabetic retinopathy fool you. It could get worse over the years and threaten your good vision. With timely treatment, ninety percent of those with advanced diabetic retinopathy can be saved from going blind.

The National Eye Institute (NEI) is the Federal government's lead agency for vision research. The NEI urges all people with diabetes to have an eye examination through dilated pupils at least once a year.

How Does Diabetic Retinopathy Damage The Retina?

Diabetic retinopathy occurs when diabetes damages the tiny blood vessels in the retina. At this point, most people do not notice any changes in their vision.

Some people develop a condition called macular edema. It occurs when the damaged blood vessels leak fluid and lipids onto the macula, the part of the retina that lets us see detail. The fluid makes the macula swell, blurring vision.

As the disease progresses, it enters its advanced, or proliferative, stage. Fragile, new blood vessels grow along the retina and in the clear, gel-like vitreous that fills the inside of the eye. Without timely treatment, these new blood vessels can bleed, cloud vision, and destroy the retina.

Who Is At Risk For Diabetic Retinopathy?

All people with diabetes are at risk, those with Type I diabetes (juvenile onset) and those with Type II diabetes (adult onset).

During pregnancy, diabetic retinopathy may also be a problem for women with diabetes. It is recommended that all pregnant women with diabetes have dilated eye examinations each trimester to protect their vision.

What Are The Symptoms Of Diabetic Retinopathy?

Diabetic retinopathy often has no early warning signs. At some point, though, you may have macular edema. It blurs and distorts vision, making it hard to do things like read and drive. In some cases, your vision will fluctuate during the day.

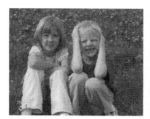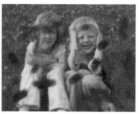

Figure 35   Normal View vs View Affected by Diabetic Retinopathy

As new blood vessels form at the back of the eye, they can bleed (hemorrhage) and blur your vision. The first time this happens it may not be severe. In most cases, it will leave just a few specks of blood, or spots, floating in your vision that often go away after a few hours.

These spots are often followed within a few days or weeks by a much greater leakage of blood. The blood will blur your vision. In extreme cases, a person will only be able to tell light from dark in that eye. It may take the blood anywhere from a few days to months or even years to clear from the inside of your eye. In some cases, the blood will not clear. You should be aware that large hemorrhages tend to happen more than once, often during sleep.

How Is Diabetic Retinopathy Detected?

Diabetic retinopathy is detected during an eye examination that includes:

Visual acuity; This eye chart test measures how well you see at various distances.

Pupil dilation; Your eye doctor places drops into the eye to widen the pupil. This allows him or her to see more of the retina and look for signs of diabetic retinopathy. After the examination, your close-up vision may remain blurred for several hours.

Ophthalmoscopy; This is an examination of the retina in which the eye doctor (1) looks through a device with a special lens that provides a narrow view of the retina, or (2) wearing a headset with a bright light, the doctor looks through a special focusing lens that gives him or her a wide view of the retina.

Tonometry; The measurement of the fluid pressure in the eye is called tonometry. Elevated pressure is a possible sign of glaucoma, another common eye problem in people with diabetes.

Your eye care professional will look at your retina for early signs of diabetic retinopathy, such as (1) leaking blood vessels, (2) retinal swelling, such as macular edema, (3) pale deposits on the retina are signs of leaking blood vessels, (4) damaged nerve tissue, and (5) any changes in the blood vessels.

Should your doctor suspect that you need treatment for macular edema, he or she may ask you to have a test called fluorescein angiography.

In a fluorescein angiogram, a special dye is injected into your arm. Pictures are then taken as the dye passes through the blood vessels in the retina. This test allows your doctor to find the leaking blood vessels.

How Is Diabetic Retinopathy Treated?

There are two treatments for diabetic retinopathy, effective in reducing vision loss from this disease. In fact, even people with advanced retinopathy have a 90% chance of keeping their vision when they get treatment before the retina is severely damaged.

These two treatments are laser surgery and vitrectomy. It is important to note that although these treatments are successful, they do not cure diabetic retinopathy.

Laser Surgery

Laser surgery is performed in a doctor's office or eye clinic. Before the surgery, the laser surgeon will (1) dilate your pupil and (2) apply drops to numb the eye. In some cases, the doctor also may numb the area behind the eye to prevent any discomfort.

The lights in the office will be dim. As you sit facing the laser machine, your doctor will hold a special lens to your eye. During the procedure, you may see flashes of light. These flashes may eventually create a stinging sensation that makes you feel a little uncomfortable.

You may leave the office once the treatment is done, but you will need someone to drive you home. Because your pupils will remain dilated for a few hours, you also should bring a pair of sunglasses. For the rest of the day, your vision will probably be a little blurry. If your eye hurts a bit, your eye doctor can suggest a way to control this.

Doctors will perform laser surgery to treat severe macular edema and proliferative diabetic retinopathy.

Macular Edema

Timely laser surgery can reduce vision loss from macular edema by half. But you may need to have laser surgery more than once to control the leaking fluid.

During the surgery, your doctor will aim a high-energy beam of light directly onto the damaged blood vessels. This is called focal laser treatment. This seals the vessels and stops them from leaking. Generally, laser surgery is used to stabilize vision, not necessarily to improve it.

Proliferative Diabetic Retinopathy

In treating advanced diabetic retinopathy, doctors use the laser to destroy the abnormal blood vessels that form at the back of the eye.

Rather than focus the light on a single spot, your laser surgeon will make hundreds of small laser burns away from the center of the retina. This is called pan retinal photocoagulation (or PRP for short). The treatment shrinks the abnormal blood vessels and decreases the eye's stimulus to develop new blood vessels. You may lose some of your side or peripheral vision after this surgery to save the rest of your sight. Laser surgery may also slightly reduce your color and night vision.

A more recent development in the treatment of diabetic macular edema has been to combine laser treatment with an injection of a medication called Lucentis. Avastin and Lucentis are typically used in the treatment of macular degeneration. However, recent studies have shown that when Lucentis is combined with laser treatment in patients with diabetic retinopathy, 50% of the patients experienced an improvement in their vision vs. 28% of the patients that only received a laser treatment.[38]

Once you have proliferative retinopathy, you will always be at risk for new bleeding. This means you may need treatment more than once to protect your sight.

Vitrectomy

Instead of laser surgery, you may need an eye operation called a vitrectomy to restore your sight. A vitrectomy is performed if you have a lot of blood in the vitreous (the gel that fills the hollow, rear two thirds of the eye). It involves removing the cloudy vitreous and replacing it with a salt solution. Because the vitreous is mostly water, you will notice no change between the salt solution and the normal vitreous.

Studies show that people who have a vitrectomy soon after a large hemorrhage are more likely to protect their vision than someone who waits to have the operation.

Early vitrectomy is especially effective in people with insulin-dependent diabetes who may be at greater risk of blindness from a hemorrhage into the eye.

Vitrectomy is often done under local anesthesia. This means that you will be awake during the operation. The doctor makes a tiny incision in the sclera, or white part of the eye. Next, a small instrument is placed into the eye. It removes the vitreous and inserts the salt solution into the eye.

You may be able to return home soon after the vitrectomy or you may be asked to stay in the hospital overnight. Your eye will be red and sensitive. After the operation, you will need to wear an eye patch for a few days or weeks to protect the eye. You will also need to use medicated eye drops to protect against infection.

What Research Is Being Done On Diabetic Retinopathy?

The NEI is currently supporting a number of research studies in both the laboratory and with patients to learn more about the cause of diabetic retinopathy. This research should provide better ways to detect, treat and prevent vision loss in people with diabetes.

For example, it is likely that in the coming years researchers will develop drugs that turn off enzyme activity shown to cause diabetic retinopathy. Some day, these drugs will help people control the disease and reduce the need for laser surgery.

What Can I Do To Protect Myself From Vision Loss Due To Diabetes?

The NEI urges all people with diabetes to have an eye examination through dilated pupils at least once a year. If you have more serious retinopathy, you may need to have a dilated eye examination more often.

A recent study, the Diabetes Control and Complications Trial (DCCT), showed that better control of blood sugar levels slows the onset and progression of retinopathy and lessens the need for laser surgery for severe retinopathy.

The study also found that the group that tried to keep their blood sugar levels as close to normal as possible had much less eye, kidney, and nerve disease. This level of blood sugar control may not be best for everyone, including some elderly patients, children under thirteen, or people with heart disease. Ask your doctor if this program is right for you.

This section was adapted from the National Eye Institute information pamphlet "Diabetic Retinopathy: What You Should Know."

Dr. Richard A Driscoll

CHAPTER ELEVEN

Children's Eye Care

Most of us would agree that our eyesight is our most precious sense, yet we often think our children's vision is fine because they are not complaining, they seem to act like they see well or "they passed their school eye exam." In 2004 the Vision Council of America estimated that the rate of undetected vision problems in children was 25%.

Safeguarding Your Child's Vision

Eighty percent of what students learn is through vision, yet 86% of all children have not had a complete eye examination . . . ever. Here we will discuss why and how to safeguard our child's vision. We will discuss why routine eye exams are important, why early detection is important, what are the essentials of an eye exam, and when should children have their first eye exam.

My Child Sees Fine. Why Does She Need an Eye Exam?

As parents, we often think that our son or daughter has good vision and therefore does not need an eye exam. Common misperceptions of why eye exams in children are not important include: my son doesn't complain of blurry vision, my child's grades are good, or the parents have good vision, therefore the kids probably do, too.

School screenings don't qualify as an eye exam. While an essential part of protecting the visual and physical health of our children, school screenings were never intended to replace a professional eye exam. School screenings prevent children from "falling between the ' cracks" and are best used to supplement regular eye care.

Because we have two eyes, it is not uncommon for children and adults alike to function normally even though the vision is poor in one eye, yet perfectly normal in the other. In essence, one eye is carrying the burden for both. If left uncorrected, this problem can lead to amblyopia, an often permanent but preventable condition, where even with glasses or contact lenses the vision cannot be improved to that of the "good" eye.

Early detection is key. It is often said that it is easier to prevent something than to fix it once it has occurred. This is especially true in eye care.

Early detection is also important in fixing problems directly related to the health of the eyes, such as retinal holes or tears. Children are active, and trauma to the eye can cause retinal problems. A dilated eye exam or an **opto**map® Retinal Exam are helpful in detecting these problems. Amblyopia is the best example of why prevention is important.

What is Amblyopia?

Amblyopia is where the best corrected vision in one eye is less than that of the fellow eye. Amblyopia is preventable with early detection. Successful treatment of amblyopia is more difficult to fix the older we get.[39] Amblyopia is caused by a big difference in prescription between the eyes, by an eye that turns in or out, or by something blocking the vision, such as a cataract. For more information on amblyopia and lazy eye see page 206.

How Often Should I Have My Child's Eyes Examined?

In 2002 the American Public Health Association (APHA) issued a statement supporting regular eye exams in children to improve the detection rate of vision problems. Instead of regular screenings, APHA recommended eye exams at age six months, two years and four years. A failure of the current screening program is the lack of follow through for children when problems are detected. Most forms of vision loss in children are preventable. Improving the access to eye care for children should be as important as are our current childhood vaccination programs.

How Can You Exam A Child That Has Not Yet Learned To Talk?

Accurate results can be obtained from children and adults who cannot communicate verbally. Rather than asking the patient "which is better?" objective tests are used which require no responses from the child. Computerized testing and a diagnostic procedure called retinoscopy can be used to determine an accurate prescription for young children. The use of cylcoplegic eye drops can often improve the accuracy of these procedures. Your child will also be examined for "lazy eye," abnormal ocular development, and eye diseases.

Frequently, the examination takes only fifteen to twenty minutes, and the vast majority of children enjoy their time at the office. Best results are usually obtained if the visit is scheduled when your child is usually at his or her best by avoiding nap times.

How Do I Know If My Child Is Getting A Good Eye Exam?

How do you know your child or family is receiving the eye care they deserve? With the advanced technology available to eye doctors today, we are able to diagnose and treat many conditions before they are problematic. Below are the essential components of a complete eye exam.

The Chief Complaint

A proper eye exam starts with what we call a chief complaint; essentially, what caused you to schedule your appointment? Sometimes patients are having a specific problem, such as blurriness at the computer, difficulty with night driving, or headaches. At other times patients present to their eye doctor for preventative eye care.

The Medical History

You may wonder why the eye doctor needs to know about the medications you are taking or why is it important for the eye doctor to know your daughter's grandmother had diabetes. After all, you are here for an eye exam, right? Many systemic diseases are first detected with an eye exam. The eye is a window into the body.

We have found that it is easier to accurately remember your health history while filling out the forms in the convenience of your own home rather than trying to hurry and fill out more forms right before your eye exam. Many doctor's offices will email you the entrance and history forms prior to the exam or tell you where to download them from their website. We find that patients prefer to enter their data at home rather than at the office, and the data collected is much more complete.

Currently, the U.S. Government, through the Medicare and Medicaid programs, is pushing doctors to implement Electronic Health Records (EHR). Most EHR systems allow you, the patient, to enter your demographic data, insurance information, medications, and medical history through a secure portal at home via your doctor's website. The information is then downloaded into your doctor's HER. This is the wave of the future, and within five years 80% of doctors will utilize this capability.

Visual Acuities

Your eye doctor needs to know how well your current mode of correction is working for you. It is important to bring all forms of vision correction, glasses, and contacts with you to your exam.

Pretesting

Here a technician will collect data for the doctor. Among the tests conducted are lensometry (determines the prescription of your old glasses), autorefraction (gives the doctor a starting point in determining your eyeglass prescription), keratometry (measures the curves on the cornea), tonometry (measures the pressure in the eye), visual fields (used to help diagnose tumors and glaucoma), and retinal pictures (the **opto**map® Retinal Exam, for instance, gives a panoramic view of the back of the eye to aid in the diagnosis of diabetes, glaucoma, macular degeneration, retinal tumors, holes, tears, and detachments).

Refraction

Here the doctor determines your refractive error, the spectacle prescription that makes you see your very best. In calculating your prescription, your doctor will determine if you have astigmatism, nearsightedness, farsightedness, or presbyopia.

Eye Health Evaluation

Potentially the most important part of an eye exam is evaluating the health of the eye. Here we can observe and detect conditions before they become problems. The eye is the only place in the body where arteries and veins can be directly viewed without surgery, thus many systemic conditions are first diagnosed in an eye exam.

The eyelids and the external parts of the eye itself, such as the conjunctiva, cornea, iris, sclera, and intra-ocular lens, can all be viewed with the slit lamp biomicroscope. The slit lamp, as we call it, is an instrument attached to a table that sits on a swinging arm. The doctor swings it into position and instructs you to put your chin in the chin rest. With special lenses, the slit lamp can also be used to examine the retinal fundus as well.

The retinal health can be evaluated in a number of ways. The most common method is via the direct ophthalmoscope. The doctor holds the ophthalmoscope in his hand, against his eye, then moves close to the patient's eye. The second most common approach is to evaluate the retinal health with a binocular indirect ophthalmoscope through dilated pupils. Often both techniques are used to evaluate a patient's retinal health.

Most patients, if not all, hate to be dilated. The **opto**map® Retinal Exam technology utilizes a panoramic camera to give doctors another option to view up to 81% the retina. While not a replacement for viewing the retina via ophthalmoscopy, the **opto**map® uses scanning lasers for only a quarter of a second to attain its images without requiring the eyes to be dilated. For more information on why your eye doctor needs to dilate your eyes, see page 201.

Having retinal photographs in your medical record can also be of invaluable assistance in your continuing eye care since it gives your doctor a point of reference when he or she needs to compare potential changes in your retinal health.

Consulting With The Doctor

The doctor should then bring all of the information together and consult with you on all of the findings, thoroughly answering all of your questions. Some of the vision treatment options available to us are, of course, glasses; however, another option to consider is contact lenses.

Your doctor will also review your ocular health with you, give you information on conditions she may be concerned about, and/or recommend further testing. Your doctor will also give you information on any conditions you talk about, provide you with additional resources should you wish to learn more, and give you advice preventative care.

How Old Should My Child Be For Their First Eye Exam?

Children should have their eyes examined at any age if a problem is suspected. Until recently, eye exams were recommended for all children before they entered kindergarten. However, numerous national organizations, such as the American Optometric Association, American Academy of Ophthalmology, and Prevent

Blindness America, have begun to recommend that your child receive their first eye exam at six months of age, then again at three years of age. Many forms of blindness, or amblyopia, that occur in children can be prevented if caught early. Before you take your child to your eye doctor ask if he is set up to evaluate children your child's age. Not all eye doctors see young children.

CHAPTER TWELVE

Eyeglasses

It is said that eyeglasses were invented in Italy during the late thirteenth century, and it is widely reported that Ben Franklin invented bifocals which allowed him to see at both distance and near. Whether Ben Franklin was truly the inventor of the bifocal lens is unclear; however, he was surely one of the first to wear eyeglasses with bifocal lenses. It appears that bifocals were invented sometime between 1760 and 1780.

Questions About Eyeglass Lenses

How Do Bifocals Without Lines Work?

It is pretty amazing how a pair of no line progressive bifocal lenses work. By using multiple changing curves, the lenses change their focus from distance to near. When looking straight ahead progressive lenses allow you to see clearly at far distances. As you look down, the power increases, allowing for clear near vision. The farther you look down in the lens, the focusing power increases, making things held close clear.

How Do Polarized Lenses Work?

Typically, light radiates in all directions. Polarized lenses filter the light so that it radiates in only one direction, with all of the light waves parallel to each other. By filtering light in this way, polarized lenses dramatically reduce reflections from shiny objects such as chrome or the surface of water. Polarized lenses will allow you to see into clear water by eliminating these reflections.

Can I Get Monovision Glasses?

"I can't wear bifocals. I want some monovision glasses like my contacts" is a common request. Unfortunately, monovision glasses are rarely successful. The problem is that they usually cause too much eyestrain and patients cannot adapt. When you see a person wearing monovision glasses, one of their eyes will often look more magnified or larger than the other.

When we see an object, an image is projected onto the retina of each eye. Our brain then takes these two images and merges them. In monovision, the two images projected onto the retina will be of significantly different sizes due to the different prescription in each lens. Our brains will try to merge these images, but experience significant difficulty resulting in eyestrain.

Will OTC Readers Hurt My Eyes?

Over the counter (OTC) readers are popular, and for good reason. Many people have good distance vision, yet when they hit their wisdom years and find themselves in need of some help to see up close, OTC glasses provide an easy, inexpensive solution. Over the counter glasses won't harm your eyes, though they may not correct your vision completely, and your eye doctor may be able to suggest a more efficient alternative. OTC glasses are one size fits all, therefore your eyes may not be looking through the optical center of the lenses, which will cause unneeded eyestrain, and you may find it a hassle having to take them on and off when switching from distance and near.

I find the biggest downside to using OTC glasses is that patients think that if they can see well with the OTC readers, they don't need an eye exam. It is not uncommon for us to see a fifty-year-old patient come in for his first eye exam and sheepishly admit that the he's been using "cheaters" all of these years, but now they aren't doing the job anymore, thus prompting his visit to the eye doctor. How well one sees is important; however, it is a poor indicator of overall ocular health. Most eye conditions can be prevented if caught early. Because the eye is essentially nerve tissue, we can't reverse any damage that is done, thus prevention and early detection are the keys to good ocular health.

So enjoy your readers, but go ahead and get an eye exam and make sure that your eyes are healthy. As a matter of fact, your eye doctor may very well prescribe OTC readers for you.

Eyeglasses And Myopia Progression

If I Wear Glasses It Will Make My Eyes Worse, Right?

No, this is one of the most common wives' tales. Wearing neither eyeglasses or contact lenses will make you accelerate the progression of nearsightedness. As a matter of fact, studies have shown that wearing eyeglasses or contact lenses that do not fully correct your vision can *accelerate* the progression of nearsightedness.

Wearing Weaker Eyeglasses Will Keep Me From Getting More Nearsighted, Right?

It is quite the opposite actually. A 2002 Study by Chung showed that when nearsighted patients were under-corrected by -0.75D, their nearsightedness actually increased at a faster rate than those patients who had their vision fully corrected.[40] The study was stopped after two years when it became clear that under-correction actually accelerated the progression of nearsightedness. What this study tells us is that it is okay to wear our glasses and we should make sure our glasses incorporate our current prescription. A comprehensive review of myopia prevention can be found at http://bit.ly/myopia-prevent . For more information on preventing the progression of nearsightedness see page 83.

Buying Your Eyeglasses

What Is The Advantage To Buying My Eyeglasses From My Eye Doctor?

There are a lot of good reasons to buy your glasses from the same doctor that wrote you the prescription. Here are the top 5:

1. You are supporting a local business. Almost all chain eyeglass companies are owned by large corporations. Half of the retail eyeglass companies are owned by foreign companies.

2. No one wants to ensure that you are happy with your eyeglass selection more than your eye doctor. In a big corporation there are a lot of layers of management. If there is a problem, it's hard to get to the top. You see your local doctor and his staff around town, he or she wants to make you happy, so you'll send more patients their way.

3. Your eye doctor's office is probably a lot closer than the local mall, making it much easier to stop by your doctor's office for a quick repair or adjustment.

4. Your will find that purchasing eyeglasses from your eye doctor is price competitive. When comparing apples to apples, the fee you pay for glasses from your local doc versus the big chains will be close.

5. A better, more diverse selection of eyeglass frames and ophthalmic lenses will be available from your eye doctor's office. Your local doctor has access to ophthalmic frames and lenses from any supplier. The eyeglass chains' selection of both eyeglass frames and lenses are limited because they are often tied into certain manufacturers.

Can I Use My Health Savings Plan Or Flex Plan For Eye Care Expenses?

Yes, currently eye exams, contact lenses, orthokeratology, glasses, and refractive surgery are considered reimbursable expenses under flex plans and health savings accounts.

Eyeglasses and Children

What Kind Of Eyeglass Lenses Are Recommended For Children?

Assessing the visual needs of your child with an eye exam is the first step in protecting your child's vision. It is equally important to select lenses that will not only make them see well, but also protect their eyes.

Polycarbonate or Trivex lenses are the only lens types that have the potential to reduce, not increase, the risk of serious eye injury. Polycarbonate and Lexan are used in bullet-proof windshields, safety glasses, helicopter canopies, and many other high performance applications. Other lens types, including glass and regular plastic (CR-39), will break into pieces upon impact. Often the impact from an object does less damage to the victim than the broken eyeglass lenses.

Both polycarbonate and Trivex are thin, lightweight, and highly impact resistant. Kids can do crazy things, and accidents can happen; therefore, polycarbonate and Trivex are not just recommended for sports, but should be used to protect their eyes every day.

Trivex is highly scratch resistant, making it the best option for children. Polycarbonate is much softer and therefore less scratch resistant; however, it is slightly less expensive and a little thinner. Both lens materials naturally block 100% of UV light without any additional coatings. The optical qualities of Trivex are much better than those of polycarbonate; therefore, there is less distortion and reflection from an ophthalmic lens made of Trivex. Both lens materials are available in Transitions (automatically get darker outside, lighter inside) and accept an antireflective coating which prevents reflections, making the lenses look transparent.

Should I Get A Reflection Free Coating For My Child's Glasses?

Everyone likes to see without reflections. Reflection-free coatings are more expensive; however, the newer coatings make the lenses much easier to clean, and more importantly, they can harden the lens surface, making their scratch resistance as good as a glass lens. This is especially important for kids as they tend to be much harder on their glasses.

Seven Important Tips On Buying Sunglasses

We love our sunglasses, but how do you know what features are important? Let's separate the wheat from the chaff. According to the American Optometric Association, the seven most important things to consider when buying sunglasses are as follows:

1. I pretty much wear sunglasses anytime I'm outside, not because they make me look marginally cooler (one can dream), but because it's easier on the eyes, and it gives me a headache if I have to squint all of the time. Don't forget to wear them on cloudy days, too. You would be surprised how much UV light is still bouncing around on a cloudy day. So if you are going to be wearing them a lot, get a pair that is light and comfortable.

2. UV protection is probably the most important feature. Look for sunglasses that are well made and that block out 99 to 100% of the UV-A and UV-B radiation. Good sunglasses will probably block out 75 to 90% of the visible light.

3. Now we know that UV protection is important in sunglasses, but so is the size of lenses. I know those John Lennon sunglasses with lenses the size of a quarter look cool and you had a heck of a time finding them, but they don't cover much of your eye. Small diameter lenses are better for activities that have a lower chance for UV exposure, such as driving where the windshield will block 60% of the UV light. If you are going to participate in activities where the UV is high such, as mountain climbing, playing in the snow, for example look, for larger lenses so your eye is better covered.

4. Make sure that the left and right lenses are the same color and density. I know you would think that this is obvious, but a lot of the cheapo shades have poor quality lenses. Hold the lens out in front of you, move it around, and see if it distorts distant objects. If it does, find another pair. Good quality lenses should also be scratch resistant.

5. Most people prefer gray lenses because they reduce the light without altering the colors; however, in some sports, different colored sunglasses are helpful.

6. Pick up a pair of shades for your kids as well. They spend more time outside than we do.

7. Sunglasses can be activity-specific. Your cycling shades may not be the same as those you use for driving or reading by the pool.

Dr. Richard Driscoll

CHAPTER THIRTEEN

Miscellaneous

This section has a little of everything. Some questions just didn't fall into a good category. I hope you find your answers here. If you don't find the answer to your questions here, feel free to visit www.TheEyeDocBlog.com and your question may be answered on the blog or find its way into a future edition of this book.

Myopia Prevention/Progression

My Child's Eyes Keep Getting Worse, How Can I Slow Down Or Stop Her From Getting More Nearsighted?

Yes, current research shows that there are a number of ways to slow the progression of nearsightedness in our children. The next few questions below will cover some of the current techniques.

Research into preventing the progression of myopia is a hot topic. Myopia prevention research is especially strong in China. The MyopiaPrevention.org website is an excellent resource for locating the latest studies on myopia research. This URL http://bit.ly/myopia-prev-references will take you directly to the research page. Orthokeratology has been proven effective in the prevention of myopia more information is available on page 83.

Can Contact Lenses Slow Down Myopia?

Numerous recent studies have shown that orthokeratology lenses can prevent the progression of myopia (nearsightedness) in children.[41],[42] Why is it important to prevent the progression of nearsightedness in our children? The incidence of myopia in the United States increased by 66% in the last thirty years.[1] The Stabilization of Myopia by Accelerated Reshaping Technique (SMART), a four-year, multi-center study, recently concluded, and we are awaiting the final results. However previous preliminary reports of this study indicated that orthokeratology did indeed effectively prevent the progression of nearsightedness.[43]

Other recent studies have also shown that the overnight orthokeratology technology effectively slows and possibly even halts the progression of myopia in children.

One such study, Controlling Astigmatism and Nearsightedness in Developing Youth (CANDY Study), showed that modern corneal shaping lenses were effective in reducing the progression of nearsightedness in children between nine and eighteen years of age.[44]

The CANDY Study involved children who wore Vision Shaping Lenses while they were asleep.

The prevention of myopia is currently an important and active area of study. Thus far the various studies show that orthokeratology slows the progression of myopia from 50% to 90%. That is a wide range, and clearly more work needs to be done in this area of research.

Does Research Show That Orthokeratology Prevents The Progression Of Nearsightedness?

Almost a year ago the study Controlling Astigmatism & Nearsightedness in Developing Youth (CANDY), showed that orthokeratology contact lenses reduced the progression of nearsightedness in kids between nine and sixteen. The authors of the

CANDY study found that the amount myopia in children that did not wear the overnight Corneal Refractive Therapy lenses increased at a rate of .37D per year while those children wearing the lenses progressed at only .03 Diopters per year.

Another study, Corneal Reshaping and Myopia Progression, published in the *British Journal of Ophthalmology*, conducted at the Ohio State University College of Optometry found that the eyes of the children wearing overnight orthokeratology lenses increased in length at a markedly slower rate than the study's non Ortho-K lens wearers.

Last, clinical trials for the multi-center, four year study, Stabilization of Myopia by Accelerated Reshaping Technique (SMART) ended in 2011. We should expect to see the final results soon. However, earlier reports from the authors indicated that orthokeratology lenses appear to markedly slow the progression of nearsightedness in children.

While the rate of nearsightedness in the US population has increased significantly in the last thirty years, it is comforting to know that there are safe and effective methods of slowing the progression of myopia.

Can Eye Drops Slow The Progression Of Nearsightedness?

Yes, we have known for years that atropine eye drops will greatly slow the progression of myopia in children; however, atropine eye drops are not without significant side effects.[45] One drop of 1% atropine will keep your eye dilated for weeks. Not only does atropine dilate your eyes, it keeps you from focusing up close, too. While successful in slowing myopia, most kids discontinue therapy after a short time.

Shortly before this book was about to go to press, a study of 400 school-age Taiwanese children was published using low concentrations of atropine to slow the progression of myopia. The study found that 0.01% atropine eye drops had minimal side effects while retaining comparable effectiveness in the prevention of nearsightedness to the stronger concentrations.[46]

I expect that it will be commonplace for eye doctors to prescribe 0.01% atropine eye drops, combined with orthokeratology, to greatly slow the progression of nearsightedness in the near future.

Will The Bates Method Really Make My Eyes Better

The short answer is a resounding NO, but if you want to learn more please read on. First, let's cover a little background on the Dr. Bates. William Horatio Bates, MD was an ophthalmologist practicing in the early 1900s. He felt that a person's eyesight could be improved via eye exercises. Bates' eye exercises should not be confused with the eye exercises used in vision training, which have been shown to help eye problems such as amblyopia and eye coordination. Bates' eye exercises consisted of

- **Palming**—closing and covering the eyes with your hands to relax them

- **Sunning**—focusing sunlight on the white part of the eyes (sclera)

- **Movement**—moving the eyes up and down and side to side

- **Visualization**—imagine something black such as the largest letter in a Snellen chart (eye chart), then visualize progressively smaller letters.

The Bates Method still has its ardent advocates, most of whom seem to be selling how to books; however, the Bates Method has been *overwhelmingly* disproved as having no positive effect on improving a person's vision.

Can Eyeglasses Prevent Myopia?

Though not as effective as orthokeratology, eyeglasses incorporating prism and bifocal lenses were shown to slow the progression of myopia in children.[47]

Defining the Three O's, Optometrists, Ophthalmologists and Opticians

Patients often get "The Three O's" confused. What are "The Three O's?" The roles and responsibilities of an optometrist, ophthalmologist, and optician are often confused. All of the "O's" are vital to providing patients with the quality eye care they deserve.

Is it Opthalmologist or Ophthalmologist, What Is The Correct Spelling?

You are not alone, many people misspell ophthalmologist (of-thuhl-mol-uh-jist), the correct spelling however, is ophthalmologist with two h's. As a matter of fact, Facebook continues to misspell ophthalmologist even into the Spring of 2012.

What Is An Optometrist?

A Doctor of Optometry (O.D.) is a health care professional trained and state licensed to provide primary and secondary eye care services. These services include comprehensive eye health and vision examinations; diagnosis and treatment of eye diseases, including glaucoma, cataracts, and vision disorders; the detection of general health problems; the prescribing of glasses, contact lenses, low vision rehabilitation, vision therapy and medications; the performing of certain surgical procedures; and the counseling of patients regarding their surgical alternatives and vision needs as related to their occupations, avocations, and lifestyle.

The optometrist has completed pre-professional undergraduate education in a college or university and four years of professional education at a college of optometry, leading to the doctor of optometry (O.D.) degree. Additionally, approximately one out of ten optometrists completes a post doctoral residency.

What Is An Ophthalmologist?

An ophthalmologist is a medical doctor who specializes in ophthalmic (eye) surgery. To become an ophthalmologist, a student will complete an undergraduate college education followed by four years of medical school. After medical school, an ophthalmologist's specialization is attained during a three-year post-doctoral residency where the focus is on ocular surgery and treating eye diseases.

What Is An Optician?

Opticians are professionals in the field of designing, finishing, fitting, and dispensing of eyeglasses and contact lenses, based on an eye doctor's prescription. The optician may also dispense colored and specialty lenses for particular needs as well as low-vision aids and artificial eyes. An optician can become ABO Certified by the American Board of Opticianry after successfully completing the additional training and testing necessary to demonstrate their added knowledge in advanced optics theory and practice.

Sports Vision

Protecting Your Eyes While Playing Sports

If you have ever played sports and worn glasses, you know the limitations in doing so. Glasses present obvious mobility and peripheral vision issues. In addition, regular glasses offer little physical protection and actually contribute to ocular damage if the lenses shatter or are popped out of the frame.

How Do You Maximize Vision Correction For Athletes

Contact lenses offer a safe, clear, and comfortable alternative for the athlete on any field or court. Peripheral vision is not an issue with contact lenses; however, contact lenses don't protect the eyes. For most sports, eye protection is important. Most eye injuries are preventable. Almost 3% of the emergency department visits in 2008 were for eye injuries.[48] There are many activity-specific sports eyewear options that offer excellent protection to athletes. Winter and indoor sports like ice hockey, basketball, football, softball, racquet sports and golf contribute the greatest number of eye injuries.

Visual Ergonomics – Setting Up Your Computer Workstation For Maximum Visual Comfort

The older we get and/or the more time we spend at the computer, the more important it is to set up your work environment for maximum visual comfort.

Doc, My Eyes Are Killing Me When I'm Working At The Computer. Any Tips?

Generally, from a visual standpoint, laptops placed on a desk, are set up rather well for the maximum visual comfort. Laptops have us looking down, allowing a user who wears bifocals to see the screen through the bifocal. Because the laptop screen is directly in front of the keyboard, the distance to the screen is much closer than that of a desktop monitor, thus allowing you to see the laptop screen clearly through the bifocal of your glasses.

A desktop monitor is another matter. Placement of the monitor is very important in maximizing your visual comfort. The new LCD monitors make it much easier to place them in positions allowing for easy, comfortable viewing. The monitor should be placed in a position typically 20 inches or more away and positioned low enough that, when you are looking straight ahead, you are looking over the top of the monitor. This last point is especially important for bifocal wearers, particularly those over age fifty who view the monitor through the intermediate portion of their progressive or trifocal lenses.

Why Is Monitor Height Important?

If the monitor is too high and you are approaching age fifty you have to tilt your chin up to focus with the intermediate portion of your progressive lens. If you are only at the computer for a few minutes this may be tolerable; however, if you sit at the computer for an extended period, moving your chin up to view the monitor spells neck ache. If you don't tilt your chin up to view the monitor through the bifocal, then you are looking through the top part of your glasses instead of the intermediate zone, thus straining your eyes. Neither option is acceptable in maintaining good visual ergonomics for any reasonable length of time.

So How Should We Set Up Our Workstation?

First, if your monitor is on top of the CPU, place the CPU under the desk and the monitor directly on the desk. Having a chair with an adjustable seat will allow you to raise your seat, thus further improving your position.

Second, never place your monitor where there is a bright light behind it, such as in front of a window. It's great being able to look out the window while working, but that bright light behind the monitor will soon have you rubbing your eyes. Having a window behind you is not good either as it will most likely cause bothersome reflections unless you have an antireflective screen on your monitor.

Third, place the monitor twenty to thirty inches from you. This is especially important if you have a large monitor. A quick word on monitor selection. Generally, bigger monitors are better from both a visual ergonomic standpoint and for better work productivity.

Lastly, a good, adjustable chair with some kind of foot stool is great.

What Are Computer Glasses?

Progressive or bifocal computer glasses are often not necessary for those under age fifty to work at the computer; however, anyone approaching fifty who spends more than a couple hours a day at the computer will most likely benefit from using computer glasses. Most patients simply leave their computer glasses at their desk. Computer glasses are progressive or bifocal lenses prescribed so that the top part is set to focus at computer distance, roughly arm's length, and the bottom will focus at near, usually sixteen to eighteen inches. An antireflective coating will eliminate reflections, further improving visual comfort.

Computer glasses not only help reduce eyestrain, but they also reduce neck pain at your desk. Numerous factors need to be addressed to maximize your comfort and effectiveness while working at the computer. Computer-related eyestrain is especially common for those approaching their fifties and above.

How Do I Know If Computer Glasses Will Help Me?

When working at our computer, we often find ourselves raising our chin to look through the intermediate portion of our progressive lenses to make the monitor clear. Tilting our chin up puts our neck in a bad, uncomfortable position. If you experience neck pain while working at the computer, you should see your eye doctor about computer glasses. Often we try to avoid the neck pain while at our workstation by looking through the top part of our progressive lenses. The problem in doing this is that you are not getting the benefit of the glasses helping you focus on the computer because you are looking through the distance part, not the intermediate.

A few minutes to read a quick email will usually not be a problem; however, the longer you spend in this position, the worse it is for your eyes, your posture, and your neck. Computer glasses place your monitor in the proper focus, allowing you to look directly at the monitor while still allowing you to view reading material at a normal reading distance.

Another important consideration while working at the computer is your blinking. When we work at the computer, we become so engrossed in what we are doing that our blink rate goes down which increases the symptoms of dry eye syndrome.

Is Computer Use Bad For My Eyes?

No, using computers or any kind of near work for that matter will not cause your eyes to go bad. What computer use will do, however, is make any uncorrected visual problems become more apparent. When we work at a computer, we typically don't change our point of gaze for possibly hours. Before computers were such an integral part of the office workplace, we would experience intermittent visual breaks in our focus that gave our eyes a break by turning the page, going to the file cabinet, or grabbing another document, etc. With computers, everything we need is available to us on our monitor. When we finish one, task the next is available on the computer. Our gaze rarely strays from the monitor. Even when we take a mental break, we still take that break looking at our monitor, checking personal email, YouTube, Facebook etc.

How Do We Prevent Visual Strain At The Computer?

1. The first is to set up your workstation for enhanced visual ergonomics.

2. Take occasional breaks from looking at the monitor. Once an hour is recommended.

3. If it has been over a year since your last eye exam, often a change in glasses is all that is needed.

4. If you are wearing progressive lenses, raise your seat or lower your monitor so that when you are looking straight ahead, you can look over the top of the monitor.

All About Pinhole Glasses

A few times during the life of my blog TheEyeDocBlog.com I've been approached by merchandisers to review or place banner ads promoting pinhole glasses. This begs the question do pinhole glasses work? The simple answer is it will make the image a little clearer and much darker. Comparing the vision from pinhole glasses to that attained by prescription lenses is like comparing your vision at midday versus twenty minutes after the sun sets. Okay, maybe pinhole glasses aren't that good.

How Do Pinhole Glasses Work?

First let's discuss how prescription lenses focus light on the eye. Prescription lenses focus light on the fovea (the most sensitive part of the retina where we have our best visual acuity) by taking all of light entering the eye and focusing it directly on the fovea. The farther the light is from the center of the pupil, the more it must be focused to allow us to see clearly. Light that enters the pupil at the center does not have to be focused at all. This is how pinhole glasses work. Pinhole glasses block out all of the light in the periphery that must be focused to hit the fovea and allows in only the light that enters directly into the center of the pupil, thus does not need to be focused.

Do Pinhole Glasses Serve Any Purpose?

Yes, in a way they do. We use a form of pinhole glasses to see if a patient presenting to the office with a red eye, for instance, can see better if she was wearing her glasses. As an example, a new patient presents to an eye doctor's office with a red eye. After we have asked the typical questions to provide some history about her red eye, we want to see how well she is seeing.

Often, a patient with a red eye was driven to the office by someone else and didn't bring his glasses or because his eye is red he can't wear his contact lenses. After we check his vision, we see that he has 20/80 vision in the red eye. Now the question becomes is the poor vision due to not wearing his glasses or is there another cause? Enter pinhole glasses, or more likely a pinhole occluder (a paddle with lots of little holes in it). We recheck our patient's vision while he is looking through all of those little holes, and lo and behold, his vision through the pinhole glasses is 20/30. It's still not 20/20; however, we now have an additional degree of comfort knowing that, if he was wearing his glasses, his vision would be normal. A pinhole is used to see if the vision is likely to improve with glasses or contact lenses.

So there you have it. Pinhole glasses, while certainly not a substitute for prescription eyewear, do serve a purpose as a screening tool for refractive conditions in a doctor's office.

Video Games And Your Vision

Are Video Games Bad For My Eyes?

This answer is debatable as there are no good studies at this time. My clinical impression is that video games are not necessarily bad for your vision, in moderation. The important thing to remember with video games is to take a break periodically, about fifteen minutes every hour.

Video Games May Help Your Vision?

Coming on the heals of the prior question this may seem to be a contradiction; however, a new study in the journal *Nature Neuroscience* found that first person action games actually improved the vision of adult video game players.[49]

Two groups of patients were tested. The first group of patients played the "first person shooter game" *Call of Duty* and experienced a significant increase in their ability to distinguish different shades of gray (contrast sensitivity function). The second group used another . popular game, *The Sims*, which was similar in its graphic detail, however, it is a non-action game that does not require precise visual activities.

Contrast sensitivity function is a measure of visual acuity that uses different shades of gray to evaluate a person's vision rather than the most common method of measuring visual acuity called a Snellen Eye Chart (shown in Figure 36) which uses progressively smaller letters to determine a person's visual acuity.

Contrast sensitivity is a much more precise way of evaluating a person's visual acuity; however, it is rather tedious and thus is more often used in clinical research.

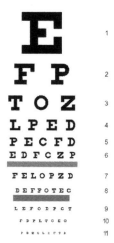

Figure 36   Snellen Visual Acuity Chart

The exciting part of this study is that it has been previously thought that it was difficult to improve the vision in adults. This study paves the way for possible new treatments of amblyopia in children and the hope of retraining patients that may have lost vision due to some retinal conditions. The study showed that not all games are created equal in producing this affect, and advised caution in recommending games to patients.

eReaders And Your Vision

Do eReaders Make It Easier For Patients With Macular Degeneration To Read?

First let us start with what is an eReader. Essentially, an eReader is an electronic book you read on a thin, handheld tablet such as for example, the Amazon Kindle, Amazon Fire, or Barnes & Noble Nook. eReaders allow you to directly purchase a book in addition to providing storage for thousands of books.

Dr. Richard Driscoll

What About An Amazon Kindle For Patients Who Are Visually Impaired?

As with most doctors, we are constantly on the lookout for items we feel may help our patients. The Amazon Kindle has been out for a few years now; however, Amazon recently upgraded the device. The Amazon Kindle, and eReaders in general, hold a lot of promise for patients who have poor vision as a result of macular degeneration, retinitis pigmentosa, glaucoma, or any ocular condition that impairs vision.

What I like most about eReaders for patients with low vision is that they use a high resolution screen with high contrast letters, black print on a white background, just like a book. However, more importantly, you can increase the size of the letters or reverse the background to black and letters to white. Changing the font size is a great option for patients with impaired vision who want to read books. The typical eReader is about the size of a paperback book and as thin as a pencil, weighing in at just over ten ounces, which is less than a paperback book.

Most new bestseller books are about $10; however, many books are available for $1 or less (many good books are even free). Amazon boasts of over a million titles available for the Kindle. Approximately 60% of the libraries in the US will allow you to checkout a book and read it on an eReader. It takes about sixty seconds to download and purchase a book wirelessly with the included wireless network (using Sprint's Cellular Data Network), no WiFi necessary. The Kindle holds 1500 to 3000 books, depending on the model, with your library backed up by Amazon, so if you have to make room for a book and years later want to reread it, you just download it again at no charge.

I also like the eReaders for patients who find it difficult to hold a heavy book or have a hard time turning the page, such as those with MS or patients who have had a stroke. Most eReaders have a text to speech option so they can even read to you. Subscriptions to major newspapers and magazines are available as well.

What Are The Disadvantages Of Using An eReader For The Visually Impaired?

The eReaders are not designed specifically for the visually impaired. While markedly better than a book, largely because of their ability to increase font size, the buttons are not designed with non-visual cues, thus it may be difficult for a severely visually impaired patient to locate the appropriate button. The interface used to buy books with the eReaders do not take advantage of the larger font sizes.

Bottom line, while not perfect, eReaders expand the reading possibilities for visually impaired patients. The severely visually impaired may find that when the font is increased to the maximum size, there are too few words on the page and they are turning the page often. My advice is to get one of the eReaders and try it out. They start out now at $79.

Apple's iPad For The Visually Impaired?

Like the eReaders, the iPad was not designed with the visually impaired in mind; however, the iPad still expands the visual possibilities for patients. I find that, for reading a book, the eReaders are superior. The iPad weights over 1 ½ lbs, thus it is a little big and heavy to hold with one hand for any significant length of time. That said, I believe that an iPad can still help many visually impaired patients surf the web and look at pictures. The iPad allows you to magnify whatever is on the screen by placing two fingers on the screen close together, then moving them apart. This allows you to magnify both webpages and photos.

As with the eReaders, my advice is to find someone with an iPad and try it out.

Tools For The Visually Impaired

Are There Any Smartphone Apps For The Visually Impaired?

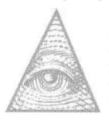

The US Bureau of Engraving and Printing has developed EyeNote™ a free, new iPhone app to aid the visually impaired or blind in identifying US paper currency. Essentially, the app is designed to allow the user to hold the bill in one hand and the iPhone in the other while scanning the paper currency. After a few seconds the iPhone will tell the user the denomination of the currency in English or Spanish. EyeNote™ can also operate in privacy mode with a different number of beeps signaling the value of the currency.

The app runs independent of a data connection. EyeNote™ cannot differentiate between genuine and fake currency. EyeNote™ works on the following devices

- iPhone 3G

- iPhone 3Gs

- iPhone 4

- 4th Generation iPod Touch

- iPad2

Scan the QR code to the right with your smartphone to go to the iTunes EyeNote™ page or go to http://www.eyenote.gov to learn more.

There are many smartphone apps for the visually impaired that turn your phone into a magnifying glass. You simply enable the app and point the camera at what you want to enlarge and, voila, there it is, nice and big. These apps needn't be limited to the visually impaired. Those of us over forty will also find these apps helpful when we forget our reading glasses ;-) .

How Can I Make The PC Monitor Easier To Read For The Visually Impaired?

There are a number of options in this regard. There is a simple, built-in utility in the Internet browser Firefox that allows you to increase the font size of any webpage and an excellent, free Firefox add-on called LowBrowse™ from The Lighthouse International.

Using a large monitor also helps by allowing you to present more words and lines simultaneously. For the severely vision impaired, highly magnified text requires a lot of scrolling, providing a less than enjoyable reading experience.

Let's start with the options native to Firefox first. You can magnify content within the Firefox window by holding down the CTRL key, then hitting the + key or the – key as appropriate to make the entire Firefox screen change size   However, in researching other Firefox add-ons for low vision patients, I came across LowBrowse™. It is a great program for patients with limited vision from diseases such as macular degeneration, retinitis pigmentosa, or glaucoma that effectively expands on Firefox's capabilities.

First of all the easiest way to get LowBrowse™ is directly from its developer, the Lighthouse International.   The step by step instructions are very detailed and easy to understand. LowBrowse™ was developed at the Arlene R. Gordon Research Institute by vision scientist Aries Arditi, Ph.D. under a research grant from the National Eye Institute. Dr. Arditi has also developed larger mouse icons which are essential to increasing a computer's usability for patients with low vision as well as improving the functionality of LowBrowse™ for the severely visually impaired.

Installation was easy and no different than any other Firefox add-on. Once the browser restarted, a window appeared just above the Firefox tabs and below the toolbars. This window is where the magnified text appears and is referred to as the reading window. Below the reading window is the normal Firefox browser window, which is referred to as the global window.

The reading window is configurable as to the size of text, font, and color. The default color of the reading window is white print on a black background. Initially the reading window was blank for me. I discovered that the Firefox extension "Tab Mix Plus" was interfering with LowBrowse™. Once I disabled the offending extension and restarted my browser, my magnification window, or reading window as it is referred to in the help file, displayed text about two inches tall.

Once you place your cursor over any text in the global window, the text in that paragraph will be available in the reading window by scrolling through it with the left and right arrow keys. If the LowBrowse™ extension is enabled, you cannot use the left and right arrow keys for navigation in the large global screen, They are only available for scrolling text in the reading window.

LowBrowse™ also has a text to speech function developed in cooperation with Charles L. Chen. I found the text to speech function to work well and was quite accurate on my Windows Vista PC. The speech function worked much like the magnification window. You place your cursor on the text you want to read in the global window and it reads the paragraph.

LowBrowse™ is a great addition to our inventory of options available for low vision patients. When combining Firefox's inherent ability to magnify the webpage in the larger navigation window with the speech function and greater magnification capacity of LowBrowse™, it truly opens up the Internet to patients with low vision. You can download LowBrowse™ at http://bit.ly/low-browse

The Secret Behind 3D Movies

How Do 3D Movies Work?

We can judge depth because our eyes are about 2 1/2 inches apart, allowing each eye to have a slightly different view of an object. The brain interprets these differing views, allowing us to note that the objects are at varying distances. Our eye's ability to judge depth is called stereopsis. Think of it as seeing in stereo.

In a movie theater, the image is projected onto a flat screen, therefore, we must show each eye a slightly different image to achieve stereopsis. This is accomplished by using either polarized lenses (the better method) or red and green lenses (think headache). Polarized lenses are by far the preferred method.

The 3D movie glasses use polarized lenses that filter the light ninety degrees apart for each eye, thus allowing each eye to see a different image. Two movie projectors are then used to show the movie. Each projector's image is slightly offset on the screen, simulating the distance between our eyes. While wearing your polarized 3D glasses, the movie looks clear and sharp. If you take your glasses off, the movie looks fuzzy, with a shadow off to one side. Your brain will fuse these views, giving depth to the image.

A Quick Experiment

While wearing your 3D movie glasses take a friend's 3D glasses and hold their left lens in front of your right lens, you will see that no light gets through. Next turn the lenses perpendicular to each other and once again you see through both lenses.

Inquiring Minds Want To Know

Why Does My Doctor Need To Dilate My Eyes?

It's not that we like torturing you with our bright lights. Dilating your pupils gives us a better view of the back of your eye (the retinal fundus). A dilated pupil allows your eye doctor to see your retina in 3D, allowing them to better evaluate your optic nerve and macula. Doctors can also see the peripheral retina better through a dilated pupil.

Evaluating the retina through an undilated pupil is like trying to identify the contents of a room by looking through the keyhole. It's much easier if you just open the door. Viewing the retina through a dilated pupil is like viewing a room through an open door. See Figure 37 below for a graphical explanation of how a dilated pupil allows for a better retinal view.

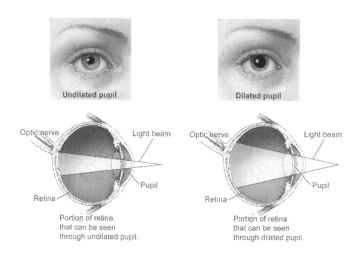

Figure 37   Undilated Retinal View vs Dilated View

Some fundus cameras can give a two dimensional view of most of the retina without dilation. See the section on the **opto**map® Retinal Exam on page 155 for more information.

What Is 20/30 Vision?

It means that an object you can see at twenty feet, a person with "normal" 20/20 vision will be able to see it at thirty feet.

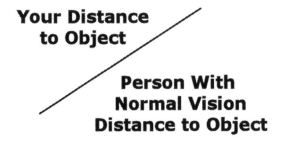

Figure 38   What is 20/30

What Are The Most Common Causes Of Blindness?

Approximately 2.75% of the US population over age forty is considered to be blind or have low vision. The most common cause of blindness among Caucasians over forty is age-related macular degeneration, making up 54.4% of that total, while 60% of blindness in African American's over age forty is the result of cataracts and glaucoma.[50]

The Police Officer Made Me Look At His Pen During A Traffic Stop. What's That About?

This is a question we are often asked during an eye exam while checking to see if a patient's eyes work together. The officer is performing a test looking for a horizontal gaze nystagmus. A nystagmus is an involuntary movement of the eye, usually a saccadic, horizontal back and forth movement.

When a sober person is fixating on an object, whether it is straight ahead or to the extreme left or right gaze, the eyes do not move. However, when a person who is intoxicated looks to the extreme right or left gaze, the eye will involuntarily start to move slightly to the left and right. It kind of quickly wiggles back and forth. This is a positive horizontal gaze nystagmus test.

A positive horizontal gaze nystagmus test (involuntary left and right movement on extreme left or right gaze) is a fairly accurate indicator that a person is intoxicated. If the officer notices a positive horizontal gaze nystagmus, he or she will then have probable cause for additional testing.

Try it on a friend after he has had a few drinks. Have him follow your finger to the extreme left until his eye has moved as far as it can to the left. Watch his eye closely, and you should see the eye quiver back and forth. Then do the same thing, having him fixate to the right. The movement is automatic. He can't control it.

What Happens To Those Glasses I Donated To The Lion's Club?

The Lion's Club collects old eye glasses from doctor's offices all over the US. These glasses are then catalogued and sent on VOSH mission trips with optometrists to dispense to patients in underserved areas all over the world. VOSH stands for Volunteer Optometric Services to Humanity.

I was lucky enough to go on one of these trips to Costa Rica many years ago with VOSH Illinois, an unforgettable experience. I hope to go again soon.

Dr. Richard Driscoll

CHAPTER FOURTEEN

Vision Therapy

Vision therapy aids a patient's visual comfort and visual efficiency. Vision therapy brings about an improvement in a patient's fundamental visual skills by improving how visual information is processed and interpreted.

Treating Eye Conditions With Vision Therapy

What Is Vision Therapy?

A vision therapy program is a series of activities of increasing intensity tailored specifically to improve a patient's visual function. These activities are conducted under the supervision of an optometrist. In-office vision therapy sessions are typically scheduled for thirty minutes once or twice a week. The in-office vision therapy may also be combined with at home activities to accelerate and reinforce the visual skills attained during the in-office sessions.

What Are Some Common Conditions Treated With Vision Therapy?

While many conditions are successfully treated with vision therapy, some of the most common conditions treated are convergence insufficiency and amblyopia.

What Is Convergence Insufficiency?

Convergence insufficiency (CI) is the most common form of visual dysfunction in which a patient's eyes have difficulty rotating inward. Patients experiencing convergence insufficiency most often feel discomfort while reading a book, doing homework, working at the computer etc. Common symptoms of CI include words jumping around a page, double vision, headaches, "eyestrain," shadows on letters, and blurry vision.

What Is Amblyopia?

Amblyopia is commonly referred to as "lazy eye." There are numerous causes of amblyopia, such as uncorrected and/or asymmetric refractive errors, strabismus (eye turn or crossed eyes), injury, or disease. Occasionally, the actual cause of amblyopia cannot be ascertained.

When the brain receives a blurry image from one eye and a clear image from the other, the brain will favor the clearer image, causing a poorly developed visual pathway in the blurry eye, resulting in amblyopia. Double vision and/or blurred/ghost images can occur, causing one to become even more dependent on the better seeing eye.

When Is It Too Late To Start Amblyopia Treatment?

The best option is to prevent amblyopia from occurring by scheduling a child's first eye exam by the time she is two years old. Early detection is especially important if there is a family history of lazy eye or amblyopia.

With early detection and prevention in mind, in the past there has been a fair degree of debate on the issue of when is it too late to start amblyopia treatment. The conventional wisdom used to hold that you must complete amblyopia treatment by the age of approximately nine or ten years old. However, results from the Pediatric Eye Disease Investigators Group found that over half of the children with amblyopia from age twelve to seventeen who participated in the treatment protocol improved their vision by at least two lines of vision.

It is generally accepted that the earlier the amblyopia treatment begins, the better and faster the results. If your child has amblyopia, I would recommend that you seek treatment for your child as soon as possible.

How Is Amblyopia Treated?

Treatment starts with a comprehensive eye exam. If a spectacle prescription is necessary, it will typically be prescribed for full-time wear. The visual pathway of the poorer seeing eye then needs to be strengthened. The better seeing eye may be covered with an eye patch or blurred pharmacologically with drops to allow the visual pathway of the poorer seeing eye to be rewired, resulting in better visual acuity.

Treatment plans usually involve having the patient wear her spectacle prescription full-time. If the traditional patch method is used, the amount of time patched varies widely from all waking hours six days a week to two hours a week for near work only. Another significant way to strengthen the amblyopic eye, with the eventual goal of making it see as well as the better eye, is through optometric vision therapy.

Studies have shown that pharmacologic patching provides better results than the traditional patch.[51,52] This method involves using dilating drops in the better seeing eye. In my experience I have found that patients much prefer the pharmacologic patching method. Its disadvantage is that kids involved in outdoor sports may experience some light sensitivity.

I've Heard That Some Vision Problems Affect Learning?

Learning-related vision problems can impede learning, reading, and sustained close work. Key factors in resolving learning related vision problems include:

- Eye teaming skills--Both eyes working together as a team following one line at a time, both eyes pointing the same object

- Accommodation--The eye's ability to change its focus depending on an object's distance

- Binocular vision--The brain brings together images from each eye into one stereoscopic image, giving us depth perception

- Visual perception--Visual memory, form perception, visualization

- Visual-motor integration--Eye-hand coordination

My Child Has Been Diagnosed With ADD, Should I Have His Eyes Checked, Too?

Yes! Children with learning disabilities demonstrate an inability to sustain near work and are often misdiagnosed with ADD when they truly have a learning related visual problem. With the optometrist, psychologist, teacher, and parent working as a team, a proper diagnosis can be made resulting in an efficient treatment plan. It has been my experience that reading teachers are good about seeking referrals for their students. When reading teachers notice a problem, one of the first things they want to have evaluated is the student's eyes.

How Does Vision Therapy Improve Learning?

Vision therapy ensures that the visual system, an integral part of learning, is working efficiently. Vision Therapy greatly improves those visual skills that promote proper learning, reading, and visual efficiency.

Seventeen Essential Skills for Good Vision

There is more to good vision than 20/20

Seeing 20/20 is not good enough. Many people equate good vision with seeing well. The College of Optometrists in Visual Development (COVD) has performed numerous studies to indicate seventeen visual skills needed for reading, learning, sports, and . . . life! It has become an assumption that seeing 20/20 is the only visual goal that needs to be reached. Seeing 20/20 is important; however, visual acuity is only one of the seventeen visual skills. Here are the Seventeen Essential Visual Skills for good vision from the College of Optometrists in Visual Development.

1. Eye movement control--conscious ability to move both eyes in a certain direction

2. Simultaneous focus at distance--both eyes able to focus simultaneously on an object/area in the distance

3. Sustaining focus at distance--both eyes maintaining the focus of an object/area in the distance

4. Simultaneous focus at near--both eyes being able to focus at the same time at an object/area at near

5. Sustaining focus at near--both eyes maintaining the focus of an object/area at near

6. Simultaneous eye alignment at distance--both eyes simultaneously directed at an object in the distance

7. Sustaining eye alignment at distance--the ability to keep both eyes looking at the same object in the distance

8. Simultaneous eye alignment at near--both eyes looking at the same object at near

9. Sustaining eye alignment at near--ability to keep both eyes looking at the same object at near

10. Central visual acuity--a measure of how small of an object a person can see at a given distance

11. Peripheral vision--area visible to the eyes outside of central vision

12. Depth awareness--the ability to judge distances or depth; ability to perceive distances between objects in three dimensions

13. Color perception--ability to perceive and distinguish different colors, most notably red, green, yellow, blue

14. Gross visual-motor skills (eye/hand coordination) --one's ability to control large muscles of the body for activities such as pointing at an object, catching or throwing a ball, stepping over an obstacle, etc.

15. Fine visual-motor skills (eye/hand coordination) --one's ability to control small muscles of the body, such as hands and fingers, while writing or drawing etc.

16. Visual Perception--ability to interpret information derived from the eyes relative to a person's surroundings

17. Visual integration--ability to integrate information from the eyes with the other senses; also, the tying together of multiple visual skills

A comprehensive eye exam is the first step in assessing your visual and ocular health, both of which are essential to good vision. A visual skills examination takes an eye exam a step further, focusing only the visual system to determine which, if any, of those seventeen areas need to be addressed and is the basis for the development of a customized vision therapy treatment plan.

ADDENDUM

Dr. Diana Driscoll wrote this next chapter on the ocular complications of Ehlers-Danlos Syndrome (EDS). She has done a ton of innovative research on EDS, much of which you can find on www.Prettyill.com. We currently have a number of clinical trials underway regarding EDS and Multiple Sclerosis as well.

What Are The Ocular Complications Of Ehlers-Danlos Syndrome

By Dr. Diana Driscoll

There is an amazing amount of collagen in the eye (80% of ocular structures), but relatively, a surprising lack of vision threatening Ehlers-Danlos Syndrome (EDS) related effects. EDS patients often manifest numerous ocular symptoms. It is important to understand which symptoms may be indicative of an urgent condition and which are merely annoying. Additionally, it can be difficult to know when a symptom is EDS related or is an indication of a non-EDS condition.

This summary should help guide both patient and doctor with many pieces of the ocular puzzle, guiding both toward conservative, but not unnecessary, treatment and testing.[53]

An incredible 27 different genes are responsible for making the collagen in the structures of the eye.[54] The category of EDS that most greatly affects the eye is the rare Type VI-Kyphoscoliosis Type. In this type, there is a lack of Lysyl Hydroxylase, making the eye structure weak.[55] Thus, the eye can perforate with little trauma. Fortunately, there are only about sixty reported cases of the Kyphoscoliosis Type VI worldwide.[56]

The following are common ocular signs, characteristics, and symptoms for EDS patients. Some patients will show many of these signs and symptoms and some will show few, if any.

High Myopia

Also known as nearsightedness, myopia causes the patient to have good vision at near, but blurry vision in the distance. Myopia is common in EDS and non-EDS patients. Myopia is typically due to a slightly elongated eye or a steep cornea, or both.[57] In EDS, however, the corneas are often found to be fairly flat, meaning that the near-sightedness is due primarily to elongation of the eye.[58]

Retinal Detachments

EDS patients are more prone to myopia and elongated eyes due to the stretching of the collagenous sclera. The retina (neural tissue) doesn't stretch with the sclera, but rather gets "pulled along for the ride" and can become thin, resulting in retinal holes, tears, staphylomas, retinal degenerations, and detachments. Dilation of the eyes is recommended annually, or any time the patient notices a sudden increase in floaters, flashes of light (usually out to the side of the vision), or if it seems as if a curtain is coming up over one eye. These are the most common symptoms of a retinal detachment and may need to be treated on an urgent basis.[59]

Keratoconus

In this condition, the cornea (on the front part of the eye) bulges outward in a cone shape, and gravity pulls the cone downward, blurring the vision and making it difficult to see well with glasses or soft contact lenses. Rigid contact lenses are usually tolerable for many years. Less than 10% of keratoconic patients will eventually need a corneal transplant due to progressive scarring or recurrent episodes of painful corneal hydrops. Some new research (discussed below) may radically reduce this percentage soon.

Early symptoms of keratoconus include vision that doesn't seem as clear to the patient as it should be, even with use of new glasses or soft contact lenses. If the vision cannot be corrected to 20/20, keratoconus needs to be considered one of the possible causes. Keratoconus is usually worse in one eye than the other.

Corneal topography will indicate steepened corneal curvature, especially on the inferior cornea. If corneal topography indicates keratoconus, this is a prime opportunity to screen the patient for EDS. This screening need not be extensive, but a quick Beighton scale, understanding that hypermobility is more common in the metacarpo-phalangeal and wrist joints with keratoconic patients, is a great place to start.[60]

In keratoconic patients, one eye is usually able to "cover for the other eye" for months to years, thus no treatment beyond glasses or contacts may be necessary during this time. When both eyes are involved to the point that the patient is unable to see what he/she needs to see, then other options are explored. This usually begins with gas permeable contact lenses, which may remain comfortable for the patient for many years. For more information on keratoconus, see page 51.

Treatment of Keratoconus

If the gas permeable contact lenses designed for keratoconus are not comfortable for the patient, one of the new generations of contact lenses with a soft skirt and rigid center are becoming increasingly popular as manufacturers are learning how to avoid the previously common splitting of the contact lens between the rigid portion and the soft portion. SynergEyes™ lenses are one of the most popular brands. Scleral lenses (rigid lenses that cover the entire cornea and overlap onto the sclera) are making an impressive comeback with increased comfort for the patient, as opposed to the first scleral lenses from decades ago.

If these lenses are not tolerable, or if their comfort is unacceptable at any time, other options can be considered, including:

Intra-corneal ring segment inserts, such as "Intacs™."--These are small semi-circles inserted into the middle layer of the cornea, usually on the inferior portion of the cornea and can often return the patient to acceptable vision with glasses or contact lenses. They are also removable should the need arise.

Corneal transplantation (or grafting)--This may involve a penetrating keratoplasty (a full thickness transplantation or graft) or a lamellar keratoplasty (a partial thickness transplantation or graft). These transplants are generally successful (over 90%) primarily because the cornea does not have a vascular system which would normally transport the cells to reject a transplant. It is possible to see a graft begin to develop keratoconus, but this generally doesn't begin to occur until at least eighteen years after surgery.[61]

There is an exciting new discovery that could change the prognosis and lives of keratoconic patients everywhere. Researchers have learned that by rinsing the cornea with riboflavin drops for about thirty minutes, then shining UV-A rays on the cornea for about thirty minutes (CR3), the collagen fibrils of the cornea develop stronger cross-links, strengthening the cornea. This corneal strengthening is resulting in the halt and even reversal of keratoconic progression. The implications for the treatment of Type VI EDS, and the use of riboflavin and UV-A on the skin is also enticing for most researchers. We eagerly await testing.[62]

Please be aware that patients with EDS, and especially those with signs of keratoconus, are not candidates for radial keratotomy or LASIK refractive correction. Because of the abnormal structure of the collagen in the cornea, the patients are more prone to poor healing, corneal ectasias (bulging of the corneas after surgery), and a disappointing result. Corneal topography or Orbscan and pachymetry results usually indicate areas of corneal thinning (prior to surgery).

Although previous studies have indicated that the population of EDS patients rarely shows keratoconus, the corollary indicates the opposite. Approximately 40% of keratoconus patients have been shown to have EDS.[63] For more information on the treatment and diagnosis of keratoconus, see page 51.

Blue Sclera

This is a fairly subjective finding, but EDS patients tend to have thin scleras (the underlying "white part" of the eye). Thus, the darker underlying layer, the choroid, shines through with a blue-grey tinge. Most children normally have bluish scleras, but as we age, the sclera thickens. This is easiest to see in a dim room with a bright light shining on the temporal cornea (while the patient looks nasally).[64]

Lens Subluxation

This is most commonly seen in Marfan's syndrome or in EDS patients with marfanoid phenotype (appearance), or those with EDS Type VI. The intra-ocular lens of the eye is held in place by thin zonules that break easily in Marfan's syndrome and cause the lens to subluxate or "move out of position." If this happens, the patient may notice double vision out of that eye. Treatment involves surgically removing the dislocated lens with as little trauma to the eye as possible.[65]

Angioid Streaks

Angioid streaks can be seen during ophthalmoscopy (best seen through dilated pupils with the binocular indirect ophthalmoscope), and are seen in some EDS patients and patients with other conditions such as thalassemia, sickle cell anemia, Paget Disease of Bone, tumoral calcinosis, hyperphosphatemia, lead poisoning and PXE (pseudoxanthoma elasticum).[66]

Angioid streaks can be easily overlooked if the eye is examined with too much magnification. Angioid streaks appear as muddy cracks in the fundus. These are actually breaks in one of the layers of connective tissue in the eye (Bruch's membrane). If angioid streaks are seen on examination, the search should begin for a systemic cause.[67] Generally, the streaks themselves are harmless. They should be monitored on an annual basis to check for abnormal blood vessel formation in the cracks which may need to be treated with a laser. Otherwise, they are mainly an indication of a systemic irregularity such as EDS, causing the condition.[68]

Epicanthal Folds

Epicanthal folds are often recorded in the literature as a frequent sign of EDS; however, a study of the literature reveals that "epicanthal folds" are often misdiagnosed, and true epicanthal folds are actually fairly rare in EDS.

An epicanthal fold is a fold of skin that comes down across the inner angle (canthus) of the eye. The epicanthal fold is fairly common in children with Down's Syndrome, and many healthy babies and toddlers have epicanthal folds that they typically outgrow by the age of three to five years. True epicanthal folds sometimes make it appear as if the child has "crossed eyes." This is easily differentiated from esotropia by gently pinching back the skin near the nose and verifying that the child's eyes are tracking properly.

What is common in the eyes and lids of EDS patients, however, is redundant skin on the upper lids, easy eversion of the upper eyelids and downward slanting eyes (the temporal portion of the eyelids slant down a bit). Again, perfectly harmless, but this appearance can be another piece of the puzzle for the doctor.[69]

Dry Eyes

Dry eyes are a common finding in EDS patients (and not uncommon in non-EDS patients, frankly). There are numerous effective treatments and medications for this symptom, which can become debilitating in some patients if left untreated.

First, the eye doctor will need to determine why the eyes are dry and ironically, the patient's main complaint may be watery eyes due to reflex tearing from the keratitis caused by the corneal dryness. Unfortunately, reflex tears do not contain the lubricating components of normal tears, thus provide no therapeutic benefit to the patient.

Normal tears that cover the corneal surface are comprised of three basic components:

The lipid, or oil component--the outer layer of the tear film which helps prevent the lacrimal layer beneath it from evaporating or overflowing onto the lower eyelid.

The lacrimal, or watery component--provides the bulk of the tears and contains salts, proteins, and an enzyme called lysozyme that protects and nourishes the eye.

The mucoid, or mucus component--the bottom (base) layer of tears. This component tends to cause the tears to adhere to the eye and prevents evaporation.

All three components of the tears in proper balance are necessary for effective lubrication.

A complete dry-eye work-up is needed to determine the cause of the dryness, thus the effective treatment. Fluorescein, together with other dyes (lysamine green or rose bengal) will indicate the extent of cell dryness and damage. A Schirmer Test can measure the lacrimal ("watery") tear production, usually performed with anesthetic over five minutes. For more information on Dry Eye Syndrome, see page 42.

Treatment of Dry Eye Syndrome

Treatment of dry eye syndrome primarily consists of one or more of the following; medications, nutritional supplements, artificial tears and punctal occlusion. Dry eye therapy must be tailored to the specific cause of the patient's symptoms. Often a stepwise approach for dry eye treatment is beneficial.

Medications

The prescription medication Restasis can help eyes increase tear production by reducing inflammation in the lacrimal gland. A topical steroid drop can reduce the inflammation that often results from a chronic dry eye (this is usually used initially, then tapered and discontinued as symptoms improve). Equally important is the avoidance of medications that can cause or exacerbate dry eyes such as antihistamines, decongestants, and diuretics.

Another treatment option is the use of LACRISERT®, tiny discs made of hydroxypropyl cellulose inserted by the patient into the inferior cul-de-sac of the lower lid. These small discs "melt" throughout the day, providing a continuous source of moisture for the patient.

Ointments

Ointments at night-time can be used (non-preserved ointments are preferred), and are especially helpful if the patient does not sleep with her eyes completely closed ("nocturnal lagophthalmus," a fairly common condition). It is also recommended that the patient sleep with the ceiling fan off.

Essential Omega-3 Fatty Acids

A critical aspect of dry eye treatment involves the use of the essential fatty acids, also known as the Omega-3 fatty acids. Eicosapentaenoic acid and docosahexaenoic acid, more commonly known as EPA and DHA, are the essential fatty acids known to improve the tear break up time by making the tears oily, thus decreasing their evaporation rate. For more information on how to choose an Omega-3 fish oil supplement, see page 61.

Punctal Occlusion

Punctal plugs are effective in retaining the patient's own tears. These silicone plugs are painlessly inserted into the lower, and sometimes the upper and lower, puncta; the opening of the tear drain, if you will. It is similar to putting a cork in the drain of your sink. These plugs are also removable, should they cause the retention of too many tears. It is generally not advisable for EDS patients to have their puncta surgically closed because of the risk of poor healing and the common reopening of the surgically closed puncta.

There is no evidence in the literature that indicates a loss of reflex tearing with EDS.[70]

Glaucoma

In glaucoma, the drainage of aqueous humor (the liquid in the front part of the eye) is inefficient or the eye produces fluid too quickly to drain effectively. This causes pressure on many structures of the eye, including the optic nerve. The damaged optic nerve can result in blindness if not treated. The most common type of glaucoma is called "primary open angle glaucoma," or "POAG." In cases of POAG, the drainage canal for ocular fluid appears to be open.

A highly nearsighted individual has a greater risk association with POAG, and nearsightedness is more common with EDS. The elongated eyeball, characteristic of nearsightedness, allows a larger optic channel with the optic nerve fiber becoming more susceptible to pressure and injury.[71]

Glaucoma can be congenital, for example, when the ducts responsible for fluid drainage fail to form completely. Some infants are born with defects in the angle of the eye that slow the normal drainage of aqueous humor, a condition most often correctable with surgery if discovered early enough. This is often seen in Type VI EDS, in conjunction with an abnormally small cornea ("microcornea") and the thin, blue sclera.

Individuals who have either Ehlers-Danlos syndrome or Marfan's syndrome, a condition characterized by elongation of the bones, appear to have a higher association with glaucoma.

Treatment for glaucoma (POAG) begins with eye drops and/or, less commonly, pills to lower the pressure. If the glaucoma is due to a defect in the drainage canal, argon laser surgery is usually indicated to open a few areas for the fluid to drain. As in any surgical treatment for EDS patients, special care is taken to traumatize the eye as little as possible.[72]

Symptoms of POAG don't appear until it may be too late to save the vision in that eye, thus annual comprehensive eye exams and early treatment, when warranted, are the best ways to thwart glaucoma and its damaging ocular effects.[73] For more information on glaucoma, see page 142.

Strabismus

Strabismus (crossed eyes or an eye drifting outwards, upwards, or downwards) can also be found in EDS patients and non-EDS patients.

Strabismus occurs when the six extra-ocular muscles that control eye movement are not in balance. Not dissimilar to the loose joints in the EDS patient, one or more of the extra-ocular muscles is looser than the others, resulting in the eye drifting or crossing.

Extra effort may be needed to keep proper alignment of the eyes, causing eye fatigue. Multifocal lenses (bifocals or trifocals) can help balance the muscle activity associated with changing focus from far away to close up and back to distance. Prism in prescription glasses can be helpful in directing light to the correct spot on the retina, so that the eyes do not need to work so hard to do so. Surgical repair of a strabismus may be complicated because sutures may be difficult to place in the typically thinned sclera of an EDS patient, especially in Type VI. As in any muscle or ligament surgery on the EDS patient, some surgical results may not have lasting effects.[74]

Macular Degeneration

The macula is the part of the retina used for central vision. In macular degeneration, loss of proper functioning of the macula results in blindness of the central vision (peripheral vision is usually left intact). Age-related Macular Degeneration (AMD) is the leading cause of blindness in those Americans over the age of 55 and it affects over ten million Americans.

The cause of macular degeneration is not yet fully understood, but it does appear that EDS patients are more prone to developing this condition. Macular degeneration can be divided into two types, atrophic (or the "dry" form) and the more damaging "exudative" (or "wet" form). Because the macula is physically supported by the collagen of the eye and receives nutrients through the network of blood vessels in the area, it is easy to hypothesize how a collagen and/or vessel abnormality could contribute to macular degeneration. More research will need to be done, however, to effectively treat or prevent this condition

A major National Eye Institute study, Age Related Eye Disease Study (AREDS), has produced strong evidence that certain nutrients such as beta carotene (vitamin A) and vitamins C and E in conjunction with zinc and Omega – 3 fatty acids may help prevent or slow progression of dry macular degeneration.[75]

Until recently, the only available treatment to seal leaking vessels in the exudative form of macular degeneration was with laser photocoagulation.[76] This was followed by Photodynamic Therapy (PDT) with Visudyne® (a drug injected intravenously and used to help direct the laser to the affected area) and is not suitable for all types of lesions.[77]

Recently, it was discovered that there is a protein in the eye which encourages the development of blood vessels. Given the name "vascular endothelial growth factor" (VEGF), researchers have been working to develop treatments to inhibit VEGF by trapping it or preventing it from binding with elements which will stimulate growth. Chemically synthesized short strands of RNA (nucleic acid) called "aptamers" prevent the binding of VEGF to its receptor. Presently three types of VEGF inhibitors are in use Lucentis, Macugen, and Avastin. All are given by intra-ocular injection.[78] More information on macular degeneration can be found on page 127.

Posterior Staphyloma

Because of the inherent weakness of the sclera in EDS, these patients are more susceptible to developing posterior staphylomas. This is usually seen in conjunction with high myopia. Binocular indirect ophthalmoscopy or fundus photography are both good screening tools for staphylomas.[79]

Carotid-Cavernous Sinus Fistulas

A carotid-cavernous sinus fistula is the rupture of a blood vessel that subsequently bleeds into a sinus cavity and/or some part of the eye. The blood flow can cause serious structural damage to the eye and is considered a true emergency. Individuals often report hearing their pulse in their temple and having a frontal headache on one side or the other. Sometimes the eye on that side is proptotic (it seems to be more prominent or stick out more than the other eye) and it can become red.[80]

Check for carotid-cavernous sinus fistula by placing a stethoscope over the patient's temple and listen for a 'whooshing' sound. Carotid-cavernous sinus fistulas are more commonly found in the vascular form of EDS, (Type IV), but all types and the normal population are susceptible as well.[81]

What Are The Ocular Symptoms Associated With Ehlers-Danlos Syndrome?

- Blurred vision that comes and goes; difficulty in accommodation

- Diplopia (double vision), out of one eye, or with both eyes open

- "Photophobia" (light sensitivity)

- Complete, or almost complete, loss of vision in one eye that lasts a few minutes; migraine auras, scintillating scotomas

- Dry eyes

- Tunnel vision

- Floaters (EDS patients have more floaters than the general population.)

- Flashes of light or a curtain over their vision

- Vision that is not fully correctable with glasses or soft contact lenses. (Doctors should perform corneal topography on all patients with unexplained blurred vision.)

- Myopia (nearsightedness) that increases quickly

Doctors and EDS patients must not assume that their symptoms are always due to their EDS and are therefore unactionable. For example, even among the EDS population, the number one cause of fluctuating vision is diabetes.

Dr. Richard Driscoll

COMPLETE LIST OF QUESTIONS

TABLE OF FIGURES

All Figures contained within *An Eye Doctor Answers* are credited to the author Richard A. Driscoll, O.D. which holds the exclusive copyright with the exception of Figures 1, 7, and 12 which are in the public domain and Figures 30, 32, and 37 which are courtesy of the National Eye Institue, National Institutes of Health.

INDEX

learning-related vision problems, 207

Lexan, 177

Lion's Club, 203

low vision, 141

LowBrowse™, 197, 198, 199

Lucentis, 136, 137, 161, 221

Lumigan. See Bimatoprost

lutein, 66, 67, 68, 131

Macugen, 136, 221

macula, 109, 121, 122, 128, 129, 130, 131, 158, 201, 220, 221

macular degeneration, 61, 62, 66, 67, 127, 128, 129, 130, 132, 133, 134, 135, 136, 137, 139, 161, 169, 194, 198, 202, 220, 221

macular edema, 161

Marfan's Syndrome, 53

marijuana, 154

medical history, 168

meibomitis, 28, 32, 48

microcornea, 219

microkeratome, 104

monovision, 74, 99

monovision glasses, 174

myopia, 19, 20, 223

myopia prevention, 181, 183

Naphcon, 36

narrow angle glaucoma, 153

nearsighted, 19, 20, 21, 102, 123, 175, 181

Nook, 193

nystagmus, 202

OCT. See optical coherence tomography

Ocular Hypertension Treatment Study, 148

Omega-3, 47, 49, 61, 63, 65, 67

ophthalmologist, 186

optic nerve, 121, 122

optical coherence tomography, 134, 154

optician, 186

optomap®, 155, 157, 166, 169, 170, 202

optometrist, 103, 185

Ortho-K. See Orthokeratology

orthokeratology, 85, 86, 88, 89, 96, 111, 182, 183, 184

osteogenesis imperfecta, 53

OTC readers, 174

pachymetry, 148

palming, 184

pan retinal photocoagulation, 161

patching, 207

penetrating keratoplasty, 56, 214

Photo Refractive Keratectomy. See PRK

photodynamic therapy, 136, 221

photophobia, 223

photoreceptor, 121, 130

pinguecula, 37, 76

pinhole glasses, 190, 191, 192

pink eye, 37

polarized lenses, 173, 199

polycarbonate, 177

posterior staphyloma, 212, 222

posterior vitreous detachment, 123

presbyopia, 24, 73, 99

prevent nearsightedness, 21

prevention of myopia, 182

primary open angle glaucoma. See glaucoma

PRK, 45, 55, 84, 85, 86, 87, 95, 96, 97, 100, 104, 105, 106, 110, 112

progressive lenses, 119, 173, 189, 190

proliferative diabetic retinopathy, 161

prosthetic contact lens, 75

PRP. See pan retinal photocoagulation

pterygium, 58, 59, 118

punctal occlusion, 48

ABOUT THE AUTHOR

Dr. Richard Driscoll, is a therapeutic optometrist and optometric glaucoma specialist. He received his Doctor of Optometry degree in 1988 from the Illinois College of Optometry. Following his graduation from Optometry School he was accepted into the 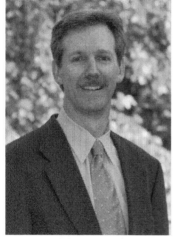 Hospital Based Optometry Residency program at the Tuscaloosa VA Medical Center in Tuscaloosa, Alabama. Only 10% of the graduating optometrists are accepted into residency programs nationwide.

Prior to moving to the Dallas Fort Worth Metroplex Dr. Driscoll was the optometric director of a large eye care referral center. In 1995 Dr. Driscoll, and his wife, Dr. Diana Driscoll moved to Colleyville, Texas where they opened Total Eye Care. Dr. Driscoll has authored numerous professional articles and has lectured on eye care technology and practice management throughout the United States. He has been practicing optometrist in Texas Since 1989. You can find Dr. Driscoll online at www.TheEyeDocBlog.com and www.TotalEyeCare.com.

Dr. Richard Driscoll

REFERENCES

[1] Vitale S, Sperduto RD, Ferris FL. Increased Prevalence of Myopia in the United States Between 1971-1972 and 1999-2004. Arch Ophthalmol. 2009;127(12):1632-1639. archopht.ama-assn.org/cgi/content/full/127/12/1632

[2] The epidemiology of dry eye disease: Report of the Epidemiology Subcommittee of the International Dry Eye Workshop (2007). Ocul Surf. 2007;5:93–107.

[3] Lee AJ, Lee J, Saw SM, Gazzard G, Koh D, Widjaja D, Tan DT. Prevalence and risk factors associated with dry eye symptoms: a population based study in Indonesia. Br J Ophthalmol. 2002 Dec;86(12):1347-51.

[4] Moss SE, Klein R, Klein BE. Prevalence of and risk factors for dry eye syndrome. Arch Ophthalmol. 2000 Sep;118(9):1264-8.

[5] Galor A, Feuer W, Lee DJ, Florez H, Carter D, Pouyeh B, Prunty WJ, Perez VL. Prevalence and Risk Factors of Dry Eye Syndrome in a United States Veterans Affairs Population. Am J Ophthalmol. 2011 Jun 17. [Epub ahead of print]

[6] Kennedy RH, Bourne WM, Dyer JA. A 48-year clinical and epidemiologic study of keratoconus. Am J Ophthalmol. 1986 Mar 15;101(3):267-73.

[7] Kelly T, Williams KA, Coster DJ, Corneal Transplantation for Keratoconus, Arch Ophthalmol. [Epub] Feb 2011. doi:10.1001/archophthalmol.2011.7

[8] Wojtowicz JC, Butovich I, Uchiyama E, Aronowicz J, Agee S, McCulley JP. Pilot, prospective, randomized, double-masked, placebo-controlled clinical trial of an omega-3 supplement for dry eye. Cornea. 2011 Mar;30(3):308-14.

[9] Tan JSL, Mitchell P, Kifley A, Flood V, Smith W, Wang JJ. Smoking and the long-term incidence of age-related macular degeneration: The blue mountains eye study. Arch Ophthalmol. 2007;125(8):1089-1095.

[10] Age-Related Eye Disease Study Research Group. A randomized, placebo controlled clinical trial of high-dose supplementation with vitamins C and E and beta carotene for age-related cataract and vision loss: AREDS Report No. 9. Arch Ophthalmol. Oct 2001;119:1439-1452.

[11] Age-Related Eye Disease Study Research Group. A Randomized, Placebo-Controlled, Clinical Trial of High-Dose Supplementation With Vitamins C and E, Beta Carotene, and Zinc for Age-Related Macular Degeneration and Vision Loss: AREDS Report No. 8. Arch Ophthalmol, Oct 2001; 119: 1417 - 1436.

[12] Tan JSL, Kifley A, Wang JJ, Flood V, Mitchell P. Dietary fatty acids and the 10-year incidence of age-related macular degeneration: The blue mountains eye study. Arch Ophthalmol. 2009;127(5):656-665.

[13] William G, Christen WG, Schaumberg DA, Glynn RJ, Buring JF. Dietary omega-3 fatty acid and fish intake and incident age-related macular degeneration in women. Arch Ophthalmol. [ePub March 14, 2011] doi:10.1001/archophthalmol.2011.34

[14] Ho L; van Leeuwen R; Witteman JC; van Duijn CM; Uitterlinden AG; Hofman A; de Jong PT; Vingerling JR; Klaver CC. Reducing the genetic risk of age-related macular degeneration with dietary antioxidants, zinc, and {omega}-3 fatty acids: the rotterdam study. Arch Ophthalmol. 2011; 129(6):758-66

[15] Wu YT, Teng YJ, Nicholas M, et al. Impact of lens case hygiene guidelines on contact lens case contamination. Optom Vis Sci. 2011;Jul 28 [Epub ahead of print]

[16] Wu YT, Zhu H, Willcox M, Stapleton F. The Effectiveness of Various Cleaning Regimens and Current Guidelines in Contact Lens Case Biofilm Removal. IOVS, July 2011 52:5287-5292.

[17] Zhu H, Bandara MB, Vijay AK, Masoudi S, Wu D, Willcox MD. Importance of rub and rinse in use of multipurpose contact lens solution. Optom Vis Sci. 2011 Aug;88(8):967-72.

[18] Walline JJ, Rah MJ, Jones, LA. The children's overnight orthokeratology investigation (COOKI) pilot study. Optometry & Vision Science, June 2004 81:407-413.

[19] Schein OD, McNally JJ, Katz J, et al. The Incidence of microbial keratitis among wearers of a 30-day silicone hydrogel extended-wear contact lens. Ophthalmology. 2005;112:2172–2179.

[20] Walline JJ, Jones LA, Chitkara M, Coffey B, Jackson JM, Manny RE, Rah MJ, Prinstein MJ, Zadnik K. The Adolescent and Child Health Initiative to Encourage Vision Empowerment (ACHIEVE) study design and baseline data. Optom Vis Sci. 2006 Jan;83(1):37-45.

[21] Rah MJ, Walline JJ, Jones-Jordan LA, Sinnott LT, Jackson JM, Manny RE, Coffey B, Lyons S; ACHIEVE Study Group. Vision specific quality of life of pediatric contact lens wearers. Optom Vis Sci. 2010 Aug;87(8):560-6.

[22] Friedman DS, O'Colmain BJ, Munoz B et al. Prevalence of age-related macular degeneration in the United States. Arch Ophthalmol 2004;122:564–572.

[23] Evans JR, Fletcher AE, Wormald RPL. 28 000 Cases of age related macular degeneration causing visual loss in people aged 75 years and above in the United Kingdom may be attributable to smoking. Br J Ophthalmol 2005;89:550-553

[24] Seddon JM, Ajani UA, Mitchell BD. Familial aggregation of age-related maculopathy. Am J Ophthalmol. 1997 Feb;123(2):199-206.

[25] Klein R, Cruickshanks KJ, Nash SD, Krantz EM, et al. The Prevalence of Age-Related Macular Degeneration and Associated Risk Factors: The Beaver Dam Offspring Study. Arch Ophthalmol. 2010 June; 128(6): 750–758.

[26] Adams MK, Simpson JA, Aung KZ, Makeyeva GA, Giles GG, English DR, Hopper J, Guymer RH, Baird PN, Robman LD. Abdominal obesity and age-related macular degeneration. Am J Epidemiol. 2011 Jun 1;173(11):1246-55.

[27] Mares JA, et al. Healthy lifestyles related to subsequent prevalence of age-related macular degeneration. Arch Ophthalmol. 2011;129(4):470-480.

[28] Dong LM, Stark WJ, Jefferys JL, Al-Hazzaa S, Bressler SB, Solomon SD, Bressler NM. Progression of age-related macular degeneration after cataract surgery. Arch Ophthalmol. 2009 Nov;127(11):1412-9.

[29] Subramanian ML, Ness S, Abedi G, Ahmed E, Daly M, Feinberg E, Bhatia S, Patel P, Nguyen M, Houranieh A. Bevacizumab vs ranibizumab for age-related macular degeneration early results of a prospective double-masked, randomized clinical trial. Am J Ophthalmol. 2009 Dec;148(6):875-82.e1. Epub 2009 Oct 2.

[30] CATT Research Group, Martin DF, Maguire MG, Ying GS, Grunwald JE, Fine SL, Jaffe GJ. Ranibizumab and bevacizumab for neovascular age-related macular degeneration. N Engl J Med. 2011 May 19;364(20):1897-908. Epub 2011 Apr 28.

[31] Brown DM, Kaiser PK, Michels M, Soubrane G, Heier JS, Kim RY, Sy JP, Schneider S, ANCHOR Study Group. Ranibizumab versus Verteporfin for Neovascular Age-Related Macular Degeneration. N Engl J Med 2006; 355:1432-1444.

[32] de Jong PT, Chakravarthy U, Rahu M, Seland J, Soubrane G, Topouzis f, Vingerling JR, Vioque J, Young I, Fletcher AE. Associations between

aspirin use and aging macula disorder: the European eye study. Ophthalmol, Epub 13 September 2011, ISSN 0161-6420, 10.1016/j.ophtha.2011.06.025. http://www.sciencedirect.com/science/article/pii/S0161642011005689

[33] Friedman DS, Wolfs RC, O'Colmain BJ, Klein BE, Taylor HR, West S, Leske MC, Mitchell P, Congdon N, Kempen J; Eye Diseases Prevalence Research Group. Prevalence of open-angle glaucoma among adults in the United States. Arch Ophthalmol. 2004 Apr;122(4):532-8.

[34] Crish SA, Sappington RM, Inman DM, Horner PJ, Calkins DJ. Distal Axonopathy with Structural Persistence in Glaucomatous Neurodegeneration. PNAS, March 1, 2010 www.pnas.org/content/107/11/5196

[35] Kass MA, Heuer DK, Higginbotham EJ, Johnson CA, Keltner JL, Miller JP, Parrish RK 2nd, Wilson MR, Gordon MO. The Ocular Hypertension Treatment Study: a randomized trial determines that topical ocular hypotensive medication delays or prevents the onset of primary open-angle glaucoma. Arch Ophthalmol. 2002;120:701-713.

[36] Merritt JC, Perry DD, Russell DN, Jones BF. Topical delta 9-tetrahydrocannabinol and aqueous dynamics in glaucoma. J Clin Pharmacol. 1981 Aug-Sep;21(8-9 Suppl):467S-471S.

[37] Kempen JH, O'Colmain BJ, Leske MC, Haffner SM, Klein R, Moss SE, Taylor HR, Hamman RF; Eye Diseases Prevalence Research Group. The prevalence of diabetic retinopathy among adults in the United States. Arch Ophthalmol. 2004 Apr;122(4):552-63.

[38] Diabetic Retinopathy Clinical Research Network, Elman MJ, Aiello LP, Beck RW, et al. Randomized trial evaluating ranibizumab plus prompt or deferred laser or triamcinolone plus prompt laser for diabetic macular edema. Ophthalmology. 2010 Jun;117(6):1064-1077.e35. Epub 2010 Apr 28.

[39] Holmes et al. Effect of Age on Response to Amblyopia Treatment in Children. Arch Ophthalmol. [ePub July 11, 2011] doi:10.1001/archophthalmol.2011.179

[40] Chung K, Mohidin N, O'Leary DJ. Undercorrection of myopia enhances rather than inhibits myopia progression. Vision Res. 2002 Oct;42(22):2555-9.

[41] Walline JJ, Jones LA, Sinnott LT. Corneal reshaping and myopia progression. Br J Ophthalmol 2009;93:1181-1185.

[42] Cho P, Cheung SW, Edwards M. The longitudinal orthokeratology research in children (LORIC) in Hong Kong: a pilot study on refractive changes and myopic control. Curr Eye Res. 2005 Jan;30(1):71-80.

[43] Eiden B, Davis R. Stabilization of myopia by accelerated reshaping technique. Presented at Global Specialty Lens Symposium, January 2009; Las Vegas.

[44] Wilcox PE, Bartels DP. Orthokeratology for controlling myopia: Clinical experiences. Contact Lens Spectrum May 2010 39-42

[45] Chua WH, Balakrishnan V, Chan YH, Tong L, Ling Y, Quah BL, Tan D., Atropine for the treatment of childhood myopia. Ophthalmology. 2006 Dec;113(12):2285-91.

[46] Chia A, Chua WH, Cheung YB, Wong WL, Lingham A, Fong A, Tan D. Atropine for the Treatment of Childhood Myopia: Safety and Efficacy of 0.5%, 0.1%, and 0.01% Doses (Atropine for the Treatment of Myopia 2). Ophthalmology. 2011 Sep 30. [Epub ahead of print]

[47] Cheng D, Schmid KL, Woo GC, Drobe B. Randomized Trial of Effect of Bifocal and Prismatic Bifocal Spectacles on Myopic Progression: Two-Year Results. Arch Ophthalmol, Jan 2010; 128: 12 - 19.

[48] Owens PL, Mutter R, Emergency Department Visits Related to Eye Injuries in 2008, HCUP Statistical Brief #112. May 2011. Agency for

Healthcare Research and Quality. http://www.hcup-us.ahrq.gov/reports/statbriefs/sb112.pdf

[49] Li R, Polat U, Makous W, Bavelier D. Enhancing the contrast sensitivity function through action video game training. Nature Neuroscience 12, 549 - 551 (2009)

[50] Congdon N, O'Colmain B, Klaver CC, Klein R, Muñoz B, Friedman DS, Kempen J, Taylor HR, Mitchell P; Eye Diseases Prevalence Research Group. Causes and prevalence of visual impairment among adults in the United States. Arch Ophthalmol. 2004 Apr;122(4):477-85.

[51] Repka MX, Wallace DK, Beck RW, Kraker RT, Birch EE, Cotter SA, Donahue S, Everett DF, Hertle RW, Holmes JM, Quinn GE, Scheiman MM, Weakley DR; Pediatric Eye Disease Investigator Group. Two-year follow-up of a 6-month randomized trial of atropine vs patching for treatment of moderate amblyopia in children. Arch Ophthalmol. 2005 Feb;123(2):149-57.

[52] Burton, JK. Atropine vs Patching for Treatment of Amblyopia in Children. JAMA. 2002;287(16):2145-2146.

[53] P Beighton. Serious ophthalmological complications in the Ehlers-Danlos syndrome. British Journal of Ophthalmology. 1970 April 54(4):263-268.

[54] Ihme A, Risteli L, Krieg T, Risteli J, Feldmann U, Kruse K, Muller PK (1983). Biochemical characterization of variants of the Ehlers-Danlos syndrome type VI. Eur J Clin Invest Aug:13(4):357-62.

[55] Heim A, Raghunath M, Meiss L, Heise U, Myllyla R, Kohlschutter A, Steinmann B (1998). Ehlers-Danlos syndrome type VI (EDSVE): problems of diagnosis and management. Acta Paediat. 87:708-710.

[56] Pasquali M, Still MJ, Vales T, Rosen RI, Evinger JD, Dembure PP, Longo N, Elsas LJ (1997). Abnormal formation of collagen cross-links in skin

fibroblasts cultured from patients with Ehlers-Danlos syndrome type VI. Proc Assoc Am Physicians Jan;109(1):33-41.

[57] Curtin BJ, Karlin DB (1970). Axial length measurements and fundus changes of the myopic eye. Trans Am Ophthalmol Soc 68:312-334.

[58] Maumenee IH (1981). The eye in the marfan's syndrome. Trans Am Ophthalmol Soc. 79:684-733).

[59] Pemberton J, Freeman M, Schepens C (1966). Familial Retinal Detachment and the Ehlers-Danlos Syndrome. Archives of Ophthalmology Vol 76(6):817-824.

[60] Woodward EG, Morris MT (1990). Joint hypermobility in keratoconus. Ophthalmic Physiol Opt. Oct; 10(4):360-2.

[61] Pesudovs K (2004). Orbscan mapping in Ehlers-Danlos syndrome. J Cataract Refract Surg 30:1795-1798

[62] Segev F, Heon E, Cole W, Wenstrup R, Young F, Slomovic A, Rootman D, Whitaker-Menezes D, Chervoneva I, Birk D (2006). Structural abnormalities of the cornea and lid resulting from collagen V mutations. Investigative Ophthalmology and Visual Science; 47:565-573.

[63] McDermott ML, Holladay J, Liu D, Puklin JE, Shin DH, Cowden JW (1998). Corneal topography in Ehlers-Danlos syndrome. J Cataract Refract Surg Sep;24(9):1212-5.

[64] Hyams S,Kar H, Neumann E (1969). Ocular signs of a systemic connective tissue disorder. Br J Ophthalmol Jan; 53(1):53-58

[65] Sharma Y, Sudan R, Gaur A (2003). Post traumatic subconjunctival dislocation of lens in Ehlers-Danlos syndrome. Indian J Ophthalmol Jun;51(2):185-6.

[66] Gurwood AS, Mastrangelo DL (1997). Understanding angioid streaks. J Am Optom Assoc May;68(5):309-24.

[67] Grand MG, Isserman MJ, Miller CW (1987). Angioid streaks associated with pseudoxanthoma elasticum in a 13-year-old patient. Ophthalmology Feb;94(2):197-200.

[68] Gomolin JE (1992). Development of angioid streaks in association with pseudoxanthoma elasticum. Can J Ophthalmol Feb;27(1):30-1.

[69] Seki M, Iwasaki M, Takei K, Maeda T (1989). A case of Ehlers-Danlos syndrome. U.S. National Library of Medicine. 27(1):208-19.

[70] Choudhury R, Revenco V, Darciuc R (2009). Ehlers-Danlos syndrome. BMJ Case Reports 10.1136.

[71] Musch DC, Lichter PR, Guire KE, Standardi CL (1999). The collaborative initial glaucoma treatment study: study design, methods, and baseline characteristics of enrolled patients. Ophthalmology Apr;106(4):653-62.

[72] Higginbotham, E (1998). Initial treatment for open-angle glaucoma – medical, laser, or surgical? Arch Ophthalmol; 116:239-240.

[73] Lee D, Higginbotham E (2005). Glaucoma and its treatment: a review. American Journal of Health-System Pharmacy 62(7):691-699.

[74] Meyer E, Ludatscher RM, Zonis S (1988). Collagen fibril abnormalities in the extraocular muscles in Ehlers-Danlos syndrome. J Pediatr Ophthalmol Strabismus :25(2):67-72.

[75] Sangiovanni JP, Agron E, Meleth AD, Reed GF, Sperduto RD, Clemons TE, Chew EY (2009). Omega-3 long-chain polyunsaturated fatty acid intake and 12-y incidence of neovascular age-related macular degeneration and central geographic atrophy: AREDS report 30, a prospective cohort study from the Age-Related Eye Disease Study. Am J Clin Nutr; 90(6):1601-7.

[76] Clemons TE, Miltob RC, Klein R, Seddon JM, Ferris FL (2005). Risk factors for the incidence of advanced age-related macular degeneration

in the Age-Related Eye Disease Study (AREDS) report no. 19.
Ophthalmology Apr;112(4):533-9.

[77] Bee WL, Lindblad AS, Ferris FL (2003). Who should receive oral
supplement treatment for age-related macular degeneration. Curr Opin
Ophthalmol ;14(3):159-62.

[78] Chew EY, Sperduto RD, Milton RC, Clemons TE, Gensler GR, Bressler
SB, Klein Rm Dlein B, Ferris F (2009). Risk of advanced age-related
macular degeneration after cataract surgery in the Age-Related Eye
Disease Study:AREDS report 25. Ophthalmology 116(2):297-303.

[79] Steidl SM, Pruett RC (1997). Macular complications associated with
posterior staphyloma. Am J Ophthalmol 123(2):181-7.

[80] Gupta S, Thakur AS, Bhardwj N, Singh H (2008). Carotid cavernous
sinus fistula presenting with pulsating exophthalmos and secondary
glaucoma. J Indian Med Assoc;106(5):312, 346.

[81] Calzolari F, Ravalli L (1997). Spontaneous carotid-cavernous fistula:
correlations between clinical findings and venous drainage. Radiol Med
93(4):358-66.